Modelling the Human Body Exposure to ELF Electric Fields

Topics in Engineering

This series provides a rapid and informal dissemination of significant new work in engineering. It is aimed at high level coverage across a broad field of engineering including mechanical, civil, hydraulic and structural, as well as other associated topics.

Modelling the Human Body Exposure to ELF Electric Fields

Cristina Peratta
&
Andres Peratta

Wessex Institute of Technology, UK

WIT PRESS Southampton, Boston

Modelling the Human Body Exposure to ELF Electric Fields

Series: Topics in Engineering

Cristina Peratta & Andres Peratta
Wessex Institute of Technology, UK

Published by

WIT Press
Ashurst Lodge, Ashurst, Southampton, SO40 7AA, UK
Tel: 44 (0) 238 029 3223; Fax: 44 (0) 238 029 2853
E-Mail: witpress@witpress.com
http://www.witpress.com

For USA, Canada and Mexico

WIT Press
25 Bridge Street, Billerica, MA 01821, USA
Tel: 978 667 5841; Fax: 978 667 7582
E-Mail: infousa@witpress.com
http://www.witpress.com

British Library Cataloguing-in-Publication Data

A Catalogue record for this book is available
from the British Library

ISBN: 978-1-84564-418-5

ISSN: 0952-5300

Library of Congress Catalog Card Number: 2009930796

Printed in Great Britain by MPG Books Group, Bodmin and King's Lynn.

To Andrea Peratta

Contents

Preface

The objective of this work is to investigate the behaviour of electric fields and induced currents in the human body exposed to different scenarios of extremely low-frequency (ELF), high-voltage, low-current electromagnetic fields by means of numerical modelling with improved boundary element methods (BEM). A variety of three-dimensional anatomically shaped human body models under different exposure conditions were examined.

The background for human exposure to ELF electromagnetic fields departing from Maxwell equations and for the electrical properties of biological tissue are provided. Then, a new improved BEM approach is introduced in order to solve this type of problems. This novel strategy, based on mixing continuous and discontinuous nodes and a new analytical integration scheme for the single and double layer potentials, has helped to speed up the calculations in the preprocessing and assembly schemes with respect to the classical BEM, leading at the same time to more accurate results. In particular, the integration method maintains high accuracy even when the internal observation points approach to the boundary of the domain. The developed methodology is applied to three different case studies: (i) overhead power transmission lines, (ii) power substation rooms and (iii) pregnant woman including foetus and evolving scenarios.

In all the cases, a sensitivity analysis investigating the influence of varying geometrical and electrical properties of the tissues has been conducted.

The results obtained in all cases allow to identify situations of high and low exposure in the different parts of the body and to compare with existing exposure guidelines.

M. Cristina Peratta and Andres Peratta

1

Introduction

Human exposure to electromagnetic (EM) fields is a well-known yet unresolved problem. The increasing number of telecommunication and power systems make the problem of exposure to the related EM fields more and more important. As a result, increasing attention has been dedicated to the analysis of the environmental and health impact of devices that emit EM fields.

Either for protection from these fields for optimisation purposes or for taking advantage of their positive effects in treating or monitoring some particular diseases, all the thermal and genetic effects have to be well known.

Regarding the positive use of radiation, it was found that EM fields could be utilised for the treatment of diseases and for diagnosis. As an example, EM fields are used for promoting bone and wound healing, for treating different types of cancer to facilitate the administration of some chemical drugs or in the hyperthermia treatment that applies EM fields locally in order to kill cancerous cells. They are also used to relieve chronic pain and different therapeutic applications in areas such as cardiology, oncology, surgery and ophthalmology. In diagnosis they are used for cancer detection, medical scanning, magnetic resonance imaging (MRI), electroencephalogram (EEG), electromyography (EMG), electrocardiography (ECG), foetal electrocardiogram (FEC) and organ imaging [1].

In general, the influence of EM fields depends on their intensity and frequency. Furthermore, EM fields can be divided into two major categories: low-frequency (LF) fields, up to about 30 kHz; most commonly found in house appliances and power lines and also electrical railway system, and high-frequency (HF) fields, from 30 kHz to 300 GHz, found in various equipments such as cellular phones, bluetooth devices, base-station antennas, wireless networks, etc.

The sub-divisions appear as well according to the type of interaction and consequent effects, and the most important differentiation arises between non-thermal and thermal effects. The case in which the energy absorption is negligible and there is no measurable temperature rise in the human body, the possible effects are called non-thermal effects.

Generally, both LF and HF EM fields can be harmful to human health if certain safety guidelines and standards are not obeyed. In this regard, the governments have imposed some limitations to the authorised radiated fields by power systems. However, these reference levels are external values. They do not take into account the way the field develops inside the body, neither the environment of the exposed person.

1.1 Extremely low-frequency exposure

This study is focused on the low-frequency region, where thermal effects are not present. The exposure limit values on current density provided by the European directive 2004/40/EC on minimum health and safety requirements in the frequency range between 1 Hz and 10 MHz are based on established adverse effects on the central nervous system. Current density is limited for protecting from exposure effects on central nervous system tissues in the head and trunk of the body. This type of exposure is acute and its effects are essentially instantaneous. The limit on current density is also provided as a basic restriction by the International Commission of Non-Ionising Radiation Protection (ICNIRP) [2] and is limited to 10 mA/m^2 across 1 cm^2 along head and trunk for workers and 2 mA/m^2 for general public. Also, the ICNIRP has specified limits for contact currents. For frequencies less than 2.5 kHz the limit is 1 mA for workers and 0.5 mA for general public.

1.1.1 Different areas of research

The problem of evaluating exposure to extremely low-frequency (ELF) and their interaction with human body in order to find possible health effects has been studied during the last 60 years in different areas of research. Distinct aspects of the problem have been considered. Epidemiological studies represent a direct source of information on long-term effects of exposure. The disadvantage of these studies is that, on the one hand, they not only are expensive but also involve collection of data on very complex human populations, which is very difficult to control and in which the influence of different external effects is difficult to isolate. Laboratory studies on cells have been very important. Their aim is to elucidate the fundamental underlying mechanisms that link EM field exposure to biological effects.

Experimental studies on animals are also important. Generally they are performed on mice or rats. With respect to cellular studies, they have the advantage of taking into consideration the whole living functioning system which can respond and interact to stimulus by inmuno responses. However, extrapolation of the results to humans is not directly due to the physiological differences between species in many variables, such as different DNA repair mechanism, different metabolism responses to mention an example. Generally, animal studies provide qualitative information regarding a potential outcome, but cannot be extrapolated quantitatively. Computational dosimetry associates the external EM fields to fields induced within the human body. Additionally, they may relate specific energy absorption rate to temperature-rise within the body. In this way, limits can be set in order to avoid high fields or currents and heating effects resulting in adverse health effects. In this area numerical modelling plays an important role. However, major difficulties – as for example finding the correct physical properties of the different human tissues or developing reliable numerical algorithms capable of yielding accurate and stable solutions for large number of degrees of freedom in order to represent as much as possible the real EM thermal picture – need to be resolved and form part of many current research streams.

1.1.2 Evidences of harmful effects

Despite the high amount of research that has been carried out in this area, possible health effects caused by exposure to ELF fields are still a problem susceptible to discussion. Although power frequency electric fields that are commonly accessible to the general public rarely exceed 10 kV/m and hence the fields induced in an isolated human being are too small to produce any confirmed biological effect, concern has been raised by some epidemiological studies that link increased rates of certain cancer, specially childhood leukaemia, to occupations in which exposure to magnetic or electric fields is greater than the average, such as those originating from power transmission lines. In 2001, Albohm et al. [3] conducted a study finding that there was a doubling in occurrence in childhood leukaemia for magnetic fields of over 0.4 μT, though summarised that the interpretation of the results is difficult due to the absence of a known mechanism or reproducible experimental support.

In 2007, the UK Health Protection Agency performed a study [4] to investigate a sample of UK homes in order to identify the particular sources that contribute to elevated time-averaged exposure. They found that 43% of homes with magnetic fields of over 0.4 μT are associated with overground or underground circuits of 132 kV and above.

Draper et al. (2005) [5] conducted an epidemiological study in which childhood cancer in relation to distance for high-voltage power lines in England and Wales was analysed. They found that there is an association between childhood leukaemia and proximity of home address to high voltage power lines at the time of birth. A 70% increase was found in childhood leukaemia for those living within 200 m of an overhead transmission line and a 23% increase for those living between 200 and 600 m. Although, it is unlikely that the increase between 200 and 600 m is related to magnetic fields as they are well below 0.4 μT at this distance, a theory that accounts to this increase has been carried out [6, 7] in which also a potential mechanism of interaction is provided by the fact that the electric fields around power lines attract aerosol pollutants.

Furthermore, there were also laboratory results in which cellular damage under particular situations of exposure have been found [8, 9].

Moreover, there seems to be groups of people who are more vulnerable to EM radiation. EM hypersensitivity has been a subject of research during the last decade [10–12]. An EU project called REFLEX [13], involving 12 participants from seven European countries, was launched in February 2000 in order to investigate possible harmful biological effects of EM radiation from mobile phones, wireless communication systems and power lines. The project ended on 31 May 2004 and the final report [13] indicates that EM radiation of low and high frequencies is likely to damage human DNA cells.

The following column is extracted from magazine 'The New Scientist' [14] about the final report of the project which ended in December 2004.

> A study funded by the European Union claims to show conclusively that the electromagnetic radiation emitted by cell phones and power lines can affect human cells at energy levels generally considered harmless. But despite the fact that the study was set up to settle this matter once and for all, most experts are still not convinced. The four-year REFLEX project involved 12 groups from seven European countries, which all carried out supposedly identical experiments. Results were then compared to see if any consistent findings emerged. The conclusion? 'Electromagnetic radiation of low and high frequencies is able to generate a genotoxic effect on certain but not all types of cells and is also able to change the function of certain genes, activating them and deactivating them', says project leader Franz Adlkofer of the Verum Foundation in Munich, Germany. But the project certainly has not achieved its goal of ending the controversy. Michael Repacholi of the World Health Organisation in Geneva questions how standardised the experiments were and says the results are far from conclusive. In one experiment, he points out, two groups reported that very low-frequency radiation (which is emitted by power lines) could produce double-stranded breaks in DNA – something most scientists consider impossible – while another group had the opposite results. 'One has to question what went wrong, or was different, for them to get the results they claim', he says. The experiments carried out by different groups were not completely standardised, concedes one of the project researchers, Dariusz Leszczynski of the Finnish Radiation and Nuclear Safety Authority. He says that, despite 2 million in funding, financial constraints meant different groups had to use different types of equipment.

Following the REFLEX project final report, there were many opened questions on the influence of EM radiation on human tissues. Consequently, in this context non-thermal and genetic effects have to be well-established and further studies are still needed.

The World Health Organisation (WHO) produced a document in 2006 related to static exposure and in the area of computational dosimetry, and recommended that further work is considered necessary, in particular, to analyse the exposure for different sized phantoms, particularly the use of female phantoms is considered important and the use of pregnant phantoms with foetuses of differing ages. It is also suggested that similar studies could be performed with phantoms of pregnant animals to aid interpretation of the results of experimental studies with these models.

1.2 Computational dosimetry at ELF

In the quasi-static approximation, the electrical properties of the tissue are such that the wavelength is much bigger than the size of the body. For example, at 60 Hz the wavelength is larger than 1000 m and the skin depth is larger than 150 m. At extremely low frequencies, as has been discussed by Plonsey in 1967 [15], the quasi-static approximation is valid. Consequently, the electric and magnetic fields can be considered as decoupled. In addition, at conditions of extremely low frequencies, high voltage and low currents, the currents in the biological tissues are mostly ohmic in nature and the displacement current becomes negligible.

In this way, it is possible not only to treat exposure to electric and magnetic fields separately and to evaluate exposure at a location, but also the electric and magnetic fields may be computed separately. Therefore, the general exposure to EM fields can be calculated by superposing the results separately obtained.

The conditions of exposure at these frequencies in many situations, like power lines, are such that the sources of exposure are very distant to the human body and therefore can be considered uniform [16].

Another advantage at ELF, from the computational point of view, is that for most tissues the conduction currents are at least one order of magnitude bigger than the displacement currents. Therefore, only tissue conductivity is considered and permittivity does not enter in the calculation [17].

In the calculations, linear and macroscopic behaviours are assumed for the tissues electrical properties (conductivity, permittivity and permeability).

As the magnetic permeability of the tissue is same as that of air, the magnetic field in the tissue at low frequencies is same as the local external field. On the contrary, not only the dielectric properties of tissue (conductivity and permittivity) are very different from air, but also different tissues have vastly different properties. Hence, tissue interacts with the external electric field by modifying it. In this sense, the interaction of human tissue with electric fields at low frequencies is more complicated than the magnetic interaction. The internal problem posed by the different electric material properties of the body together with the external problem has to be solved, therefore representing a significant increase of computational space.

In this case, the suitability of the methods is then limited by the highly heterogeneous electrical properties of the body and the complexity of the external and internal geometry. The numerical methods used for ELF exposure range from the method of momentum, finite element, the impedance method proposed by Gandhi et al. and above all different approaches of the finite difference technique, such as finite difference time domain (FDTD), the scalar-potential finite-differences (SPFD) approach by Stuchly and Dawson [18]. FDTD-like techniques are widely accepted in the literature and extensively tested in numerical simulations. However, other techniques have also been used, like the Finite Element Methods

[19] and the Boundary Element Method [20–22]. Also, techniques that take advantage of the physical characteristics of the human body have been used, as the antenna model for the human body used by Poljak and Gandhi [23] and analytical methods by King [24].

Exposure to magnetic fields: For magnetic exposure, the impedance method and different implementations of the FD method have been used. As the field is not perturbed by the human body, the computational space is limited to the body volume only.

In the impedance method, used by Gandhi and Chen (1992) [25], the biological body or an exposed part of it is represented by a three-dimensional (3D) network of impedances whose individual values are obtained from the complex conductivities (resistivities only in the case of ELF), for the various locations of the body. For each voxel, Kirchoff voltages are equated to the electromotive force produced by the rate of change of magnetic field flux normal to the loop surface. The system of equations for loop currents is solved using successive over relaxation (SOR) method. Furse and Gandhi (1998) [26] developed the FDTD method for higher frequencies. In this approach, it was technically impossible to obtain results for low frequencies due to the high computational cost involved. In order to obtain fields and induced currents at low frequencies with the FDTD method, they computed results at 10 MHz and then developed a method in order to translate the high-frequency results into low-frequency ones (60 Hz) [26].

Dawson and Stuchly (1998, 1997) [27, 28] introduced the SPFD method. This method incorporates the applied magnetic field source as a vector potential term in the electric field. The equation for the electric field is transformed into a scalar potential form, which is then solved using finite differences.

The relevant feature of both methods (impedance and SPFD) is that the computational space is confined only to the body.

Dimbylow (1998) [29], calculated current densities from exposure to uniform magnetic fields for frequencies from 50 Hz to 10 MHz. Both methods (SPFD and Impedance methods) were used to compare the results.

Stuchly and Gandhi (2000) [30] performed a comparison of induced electric fields for exposure to electric and magnetic fields at 60 Hz. They concluded that the differences between results could be explained in terms of factors such as the accuracy of the numerical method, resolution, human model size, posture, organ size and shape, and dielectric properties. Gandhi et al. (2001) [31] concentrated on the calculation of current densities in the central nervous system. Firstly, the induced current density distribution resulting from exposure to uniform magnetic fields of various orientations and magnitudes was calculated. Secondly, regions around the spinal cord have been refined and recalculated.

Gandhi and Kang (2001) [32] have also calculated current densities resulting from the exposure to electronic surveillance devices. They scaled an anatomically base adult model to represent a 10- and a 5-year-old boy. They found that for the representative devices in certain conditions, the current density average over 1 cm^2 in the spinal cord and brain of the children approaches or even exceeds the ICNIRP restrictions. This is a geometric effect that happens because the brain in the shorter models is exposed to a considerably higher non-uniform fields than the taller ones. Another example of non-uniform fields was provided by Dawson et al. (1999) [33]. They considered realistic postures and configurations of three-phase current carrying conductors.

Exposure to electric fields: Evaluation of human exposure to electric field is more complicated than to magnetic fields, because the body perturb the applied field and this perturbation must be accommodated in the specification of the boundary conditions. In most cases, the problem is solved in two steps. Firstly, the human body is assumed to be a perfect conductor and the charge distribution on the surface of the body is calculated. Secondly, the surface charge distribution is used to calculate fields and currents inside the body regarded as a conducting media. Furse and Gandhi (1998) [26] used the FDTD method at 10 MHz using the conductivities corresponding to 60 Hz. Dawson et al. (1998) [17] used a hybrid two step approach as mentioned above. A low-resolution model was used to calculate the surface charge density on the body and then interpolated into a high-resolution model to provide the source term for the internal calculations which are carried out by the SPFD method. Dimbylow (2000) [34] calculated current density distributions induced by uniform, low frequency, vertically oriented electric fields for grounded and isolated conditions from 50 Hz to 1 MHz, and solved a potential equation in different sub-grids. Hirata et al. (2001) [35] calculated electric field strength and current densities in a scaled model of an adult and a 5-year-old child (18.7 kg/110 cm) caused by a uniform, vertical electric field for both grounded and isolated conditions. The calculations were performed with the hybrid approach [17]. They found that the induced electric field was lower in the child head than in the adult head. Dimbylow (2005) [36] calculated the induced electric field by ELF exposure in a female model. The calculations were performed from 50 Hz to 1 MHz for magnetic and electric field exposures and comparisons with values from a male model were carried out. He found that for external electric and magnetic fields at reference levels, induced current densities in the central nervous system lay below the recommended basic restriction for both models.

Boundary element methods: Boundary element methods (BEM) [37] have an attractive advantage for these kinds of problems since they tend to avoid volume meshes and also their formulation is based on the fundamental solution of the leading operator of the governing equation, therefore being more accurate than standard Finite Element or Finite Difference methods.

1.2.1 Models of the human body

In order to tackle the dosimetry problem, not only the fields have to be modelled, but also the human body has to be represented by a geometry and correspondent material properties assigned to it. The first models that have been developed are either one- or two-dimensional or simplified 3D symmetric models, treating the human body as spheroids or cylinders with constant material properties. Although inaccurate and too simplified, these models were used to define the safety standard and guidelines of the ICNIRP [2]. Firstly, electric field induction has been calculated on human body models such as spheroids [38], cylinders [39] and highly simplified body shapes [40–42]. On the attempt of representing the problem, more accurate anatomy-based models from magnetic resonance images (MRI) or computerised tomography (CT) scans have been used for dosimetry. Several detailed high-resolution anatomy models for the human body in this range of frequencies, analysed on different situations and scenarios, have been already performed by Dawson and Sthuchly [17, 28], Gandhi and Chen [25, 32], Dimbylow (1998 and 2000) introduced NORMAN model of a man and calculated dosimetry at ELF for exposure to magnetic fields [29] and electric fields [34] and recently developed a woman model NAOMI (2005) [36]. Hirata et al. [35] rescaled the model of a man to produce the model of a boy.

In this approach, each tissue is divided into voxels and assigned a conductivity and permittivity value. The general idea is to use the data from the cross-sectional medical images to construct a 3D voxel model for the geometry of the human body and to assign one tissue type to each voxel, generating models of very high number of degrees of freedom of the order of 10^7. Three different male models have been developed by Gandhi and Chen (1992) [25], Zubal et al. (1994) [43], Dawson and Stuchly (1998) [28] and Dimbylow (1998) [29] and they have been widely used for many calculations. The University of Utah [25] collaborated with the MRI laboratory at the School of Medicine and the University of Victoria [25] with the Radiology Department at the Yale Medical School [43]. Table 1.1 summarises the essential characteristics of the models. In the models, more than 30 tissues are considered based on conductivity data from literature. More recently, female models have also been developed. Fill et al. (2004) [45] have produced three female models of different statures. The models have been used to calculate photon conversion coefficient for radiation protection. Recently, Dimbylow (2005) [36] developed a female 2-mm resolution voxel model, NAOMI, derived from MRI scan for a 1.65 m tall, 23-year-old female with a weight of 58 kg. The model was rescaled to a height of 1.63 m and weight of 60 kg in order to comply with the International Commission on Radiological Protection (ICRP) reference for the adult female (ICRP 2002) [46]. The model has been used to calculate current densities and electric fields induced by low-frequency electric and magnetic fields. Nagoka et al. (2004) [47] have developed a 2-mm resolution, whole-body model of an average Japanese adult male and a female, namely TARO and HANAKO, for calculations in radiofrequency EM field dosimetry. The average height and mass, body organs size and shape differ between Japanese and Caucasians. Table 1.2 shows the main characteristics of the female models that have been developed recently.

Table 1.1: Main characteristics of the different anatomy-based man models. HPA refers to the Health Protection Agency former National Radiological Protection Board at United Kingdom.

Model	HPA UK NORMAN [29]	Univ. of Utah [25]	Univ. of Victoria [44]
Height [m]	1.76	1.76	1.77
Mass [kg]	73	64 scaled to 71	76
Original voxels [mm]	2.077 × 2.077 × 2.021	2 × 2 × 3	3.6
Posture	Upright, hand on sides	Upright, hand on sides	Upright, hand on sides
Resolution [mm]	2	6	3.6 and 7.2
Number of voxels	8.6 millions		
Tissue types	38	31	
Frequency [Hz]	50	60	60

Table 1.2: Main characteristics of the different anatomy-based woman models.

Model	Fui et al. [45]	Nagaoka et al. HANAKO [47]	Dimbylow NAOMI [36]
Height [m]	1.76, 1.70, 1.63	1.60	1.63
Mass [kg]	79, 81, 51	53	60
Resolution [mm]		2	2
Frequency	Photon conversion	RF	50 Hz

Shi and Xu (2004) described the development of a partial body model, only the torso, of a 30-week pregnant woman based on CT images and its application to radiation dose calculations. Chen (2004) [48] produced a hybrid mathematical model of the developing adult and foetus through progressive stages of pregnancy at 8, 13, 26 and 38 weeks of gestation. Dimbylow (2006) [49] developed a model for a pregnant woman and foetus by means of the fusion of NAOMI voxel model, with the mathematical models of the foetus previously developed by Chen. He applied the model to ELF dosimetry (Table 1.3).

Table 1.3 Main characteristics of the pregnant model developed by Dimbylow.

Model	NAOMI pregnant [36]
Height [m]	1.63
Mass [kg]	60
Resolution [mm]	2
Frequency [Hz]	50

Although the developed high-resolution anatomy-based models are giving the most detailed results currently available for dosimetry at ELF, there are two aspects that may need consideration. On the one hand, the differences encountered in the specification of the material properties data at ELF give rise to uncertainties in the inputs of these problems.

Most of the results are based on the work of Gabriel et al. (1996c) and the parametric representation by a 4 Cole–Cole dispersion which, as shown in Chapter 3, does not agree with the mean values obtained by the statistical study of Faes (1997). Furthermore, the models can only represent an individual. Although in the case of NORMAN the definition was according to a reference man, it would be desirable to have high-resolution anatomy-based models for dosimetry calculations for different types of anatomies and ages.

The main objective of this work is to develop a parametric model of the human body, male and female, and particularly pregnant woman and foetus in different stages of pregnancy, in order to conduct dosimetry studies and to easily vary external conditions and parameters of the geometry and study responses to that variations, as well as to easily conduct studies of sensibility to material properties variations. Due to ethical reasons, in the case of the pregnant woman and foetus there are no images available of different stages of pregnancy of the mother and foetus and the dielectric data is also very scarce, thus a second objective is to develop a model of pregnant woman and foetus at different stages of pregnancy and its dosimetry study.

2

ELF electromagnetic exposure

2.1 Introduction

In the last century, environmental exposure to EM fields has increased very rapidly as the number of power and telecommunication systems grew. This chapter provides information and general background on the human body exposure to ELF electromagnetic fields. Section 2.2 describes the general classification of the EM radiation according to its frequency, type of interaction with the biological tissues and consequent effects. Section 2.2.1 points the differences between LF fields , up to about 30 kHz and HF fields. In Section 2.2.2, some aspects are discribed regarding dosimetry and measured parameters that intend to correlate the doses of received EM radiation with the harmful effects and its interaction with biological tissues. Also, in order to provide medical treatments using EM radiation, the complete field distribution inside the tissues must be known. Generally, it is very difficult or impossible to measure these quantities therefore computational methods must be used to obtain field distributions. Section 2.3 provides the theoretical basis for the EM modelling of the problem of a human body exposed to an ELF field. From a computational point of view, EM analysis of the human body at ELF involves the solution of the macroscopic Maxwell equations for imperfect conductor material. This formulation is restricted in frequency by the condition $\omega\varepsilon/\sigma << 1$, i.e. up to a few kilohertz where electric fields and induced currents can be deduced from the solution of potential problems based on Laplace equation.

Proper interface matching conditions between regions of different electrical properties including air-body are provided. Finally, Section 2.4 enumerates the different sources of exposure to ELF fields and the typical levels of electric and magnetic fields that are frequently encountered under high-voltage distribution and transmission lines, near substations and in homes in UK.

2.2 EM exposure. Basic concepts

The EM radiation can be characterised by its frequency. The primary basic differentiation in the EM spectrum regarding the interaction with biological tissue, leads to the distinction in the EM spectrum of two different regions: non-ionising and ionising radiation. Tables 2.1 and 2.2 illustrate these facts.

If radiation does not have enough energy to remove electrons, it is referred to as 'non-ionising radiation'. Non-ionising radiation ranges from ELF through the very low frequencies (VLF), LF, radiofrequencies (RF), microwaves to visible portions of the spectrum (VL).

Table 2.1: Non-ionising radiation – EM spectrum [50].

Frequency range	Type of radiation	Sources	Effects in the body	Effects
3 Hz–3 kHz	ELF	Power lines AM radio, TV	Weak currents induced currents	Non-thermal effects
3–30 kHz	VLF			
30–100 kHz	LF			
100–300 kHz	LF	AM radio, TV FM radio microwaves	Tissue heating superficial heating	Thermal effects
300 kHz–3 GHz	RF			
3–300 GHz				
300 GHz–390 THz	IR		Electron excitation can occur	Optical radiation
390–770 THz	VL			
770–30,000 THz	UV			

Table 2.2: Ionising radiation [50].

Frequency range	Type of radiation	Sources	Effects
770–30,000 THz	UV		
30,000 THz	X, γ and cosmic rays	Medical	Severe damage in the DNA structure

The non-ionising portion of the spectrum can be sub-divided into three different zones. The first one includes frequencies corresponding to the ELF and VLF, where the wavelength is much larger than the body. At these frequencies, heating produced by EM radiation is negligible in comparison with other thermal processes coming from blood perfusion or metabolic heat generation. Thus, this region is called 'non-thermal effects' region.

The second region involves wavelengths smaller than the characteristic body length and heating via induced currents can occur: microwaves and RF. Thus, the zone is referred to as 'thermal effects' region.

Finally, the 'optical region', where electron excitation can occur, is composed by ultra violet (UV) light, visible light (VL) and infrared (IR) light.

Radiation that falls within the 'ionising radiation' range has enough energy to remove bound electrons from atoms, thus creating ions. This would imply severe biological damage. Ionising radiation carriers can also break bonds in the DNA. If the damage in the DNA is severe, this can cause cells to die, thus resulting in tissue damage and death.

2.2.1 Non-ionising radiation

Even in the absence of external EM fields, very small electrical currents are always present in the human body and are part of the normal bodily functions. Digestion and brain activity, for instance, are examples of biochemical reactions which involve the presence of electric fields and the rearrangement of charged particles. Several organs such as heart and muscles are also electrically active.

In our environment, natural sources of electric and magnetic fields are also present such as geomagnetic fields, lightning, sun light and cosmic radiations. Additionally, the generation and transmission of electricity together with domestic appliances, industrial equipment, telecommunications and broadcasting are all contributing to the daily exposure we all receive, resulting in a very complex mix of weak electric and magnetic fields. Consequently, the usual exposure belongs to the range of the spectrum corresponding to the zone of non-ionising radiation.

Depending on the frequency of the incident EM field, the problem can be classified into two classes: low-frequency problems in which electric and magnetic fields are decoupled and high-frequency problems when displacement currents appear [1]. Due to the high values of permittivity of the biological tissues, the boundary between these problems appears at a frequency around 10 kHz.

2.2.1.1 Low-frequency problems

Low-frequency electric fields influence the distribution of electric charges on the human body at their surface. At low frequencies, when the displacement currents can be neglected, the magnetic and electric fields are decoupled. Thus, it is possible to study independently their effects on the human body. When considering the daily exposure at low frequency, two different situations of exposure take place [1].

- Exposure to a low-voltage and high-intensity system: In these systems the main radiated field is the magnetic one. The field is very close to the source and decreases quickly with the distance, the induced currents are located and appear as loops within the human body. Examples of sources are transformers, inductances, electrical machines, induction heating systems, etc.
- Exposure to high-voltage and low-intensity system: In these systems the most important field is the electric one. The fields decrease according to $1/r^2$ (considering point source charges) [51]. The intensity of these effects depends on the electrical properties of the body which vary with the type of tissue and on the intensity of the field. External electric fields induce a surface charge on the body resulting in induced currents in the body, distribution of which vary with the size and shape of the body. If the field is applied along the vertical direction, the induced currents flow along the vertical direction through the body, which behave like a resistor connected to earth if the body is not isolated from the ground. When the electric field is applied along any arbitrary direction, the current tends to flow through the paths of higher conductivity towards the ground. Examples are overhead power lines, high-voltage apparatus, household appliances, etc.

In both cases, the strength of induced currents depends on the intensity of the external field. If the intensity is large enough, induced currents could result on stimulation of nerves and muscles, and may affect other biological processes.

Exposures to low-frequency electric and magnetic fields result in negligible energy absorption. Consequently, there is no measurable temperature change in the human body. Hence, their effects are called non-thermal effects.

2.2.1.2 High-frequency problems

At high frequencies, that is above 100 kHz, the displacement currents cannot be neglected, and the magnetic and electric fields are coupled. Therefore, the Helmholtz's equations must be considered without simplifications. Exposure to EM radiation at these frequencies can lead to significant absorption of energy and consequently temperature increase. Generally, exposure to plane-wave EM field can result in highly non-uniform deposition and distribution of the energy within the body. Therefore, the presence of induced currents in the body and the consequent heating are the main biological effects of the EM fields of high frequency. The heating effect gives the basis for the current international guidelines. However, there is also a possibility that as a result of long-term exposure, effects may occur for exposure below the guideline limits.

There are two large areas of application of EM fields which should be treated as high-frequency problems: hyperthermia therapy, and interaction of cellular phones and ground base stations with the human body.

2.2.2 Dosimetry

Dosimetry is the discipline concerned with quantification of the energy absorbed by a biological system resulting from exposure to EM fields. Theoretical dosimetry provides the link between the externally unperturbed EM field and the evaluation of physical effects produced by the interaction of the field with the body.

In this way, calculations are used to translate the field in the absence of the body to dose quantities in the body. In non-ionising dosimetry, these dose quantities can be the induced electric and magnetic fields, current, current density and the absorbed power per unit mass known as the specific energy absorption rate (SAR).

The main aims of theoretical dosimetry protection are firstly to derive external field guidelines based on restrictions of internal quantities such as SAR. Secondly, as an aid in the setting of standards to show where restrictions on different quantities may conflict and finally, in the verification that the fields produced by a particular device will not result in a restriction being exceeded.

Additionally, theoretical dosimetry findings provide the inputs to conduct further biological studies and establish possible biophysical mechanisms by which EM fields could induce a biological response.

Dosimetry also plays an important function in medical applications, both therapeutic and diagnostic. The process of providing the link between the external and internal EM fields is two-fold. The first step is the determination of the field that is generated by some source and second is the determination of the field induced within the body by the incident field. Due to the complexity of this phenomenon, it is very difficult to find a correlation between the doses of EM energy and possible induced effects.

The quantities defined to specify basic restrictions on EM exposure depend on the frequency. At low frequencies, current density is generally used whereas at higher frequencies, SAR and power density are more commonly used.

The SAR represents the power absorbed by a unit of mass, expressed in W/kg. Although generally negligible when considering ELF, the radiated energy of the EM field becomes important as the frequency increases and consequently the absorption by the human body. In tissues, the SAR is proportional to the square of the internal electric field generated by the source of the exposure, to the conductivity of the tissue and to the inverse of the density of the tissue. Therefore, the principal biological effect as the frequency increases with the consequent increase of the absorption of energy is dominantly thermal. Thus, the hazardous EM field levels can be quantified analysing the thermal response of the human body exposed to the EM radiation.

If the total power absorbed by the body is large enough to cause protective mechanisms for heat control to break-down, this may lead to a rise in the body temperature. This may cause harmful effects. The problem to be considered is divided into two sub-categories: first the rate of power deposition in tissue due to the EM radiation has to be determined and then the related temperature distribution within the body has to be calculated [52].

The thermal response of the human body is a result of complex and different physiological processes. The bio-heat equation proposed by Pennes in 1948 [53], generally used by several researchers at high frequencies, accurately describes local temperature responses of homogeneous tissues to thermal sources [52, 54, 55]. The bio-heat transfer equation expresses the energy balance between conductive heat transfer in a volume control of tissue, heat loss due to perfusion effect, internal heat generation due to metabolism, cooling of the skin by sweating and evaporation, and energy deposition due to the EM irradiation.

Table 2.3 represents a short overview of biomechanisms, corresponding dosimetry quantities and measures of exposure, which are being used in the different guidelines and standards for protection from non-ionising radiation.

Table 2.3: Biomechanisms and dosimetry parameters [50].

Frequency range	Biomechanism	Dosimetry	Measure of exposure
VLF/LF 3–100 kHz	Stimulation of muscles nerves burnings electrocution genetics?	Current density in stimulated tissue	**E**, **H**, induced and contact currents
Medium RF range (MF–SHF) 100 kHz–3 GHz	Tissue heating	SAR in W/kg	E^2, H^2 induced and contact currents
Microwave and millimetre range 3–300 GHz	Superficial heating	Power density in W/kg	E^2, power density

2.2.2.1 Methods for dosimetry

As stated before to calculate current densities or SAR values, it is necessary to know the distribution of the EM field in the interior of the body. In the case of living beings, measurements of EM fields in tissues or organs cannot be performed directly. Therefore, in order to estimate the values of EM fields inside the body indirect measurement techniques together with computer simulations are required. Therefore, in order to estimate the SAR or current density distribution in the body exposed under different types and conditions of radiation experimental methods and theoretical methods are used together.

- Methods of experimental measurement: Measurements are carried out using living animals or dummies. Dummies are artificially produced in order to reproduce the same electric characteristics of real tissues.
- Methods of theoretical dosimetry: The aim of theoretical methods is to create models that simulate the EM problem. By solving Maxwell equations, the electric and magnetic field can be found inside the human body and consequently derived the current density or SAR. A combination of techniques has been used to calculate the fields induced within the human body depending on the frequency of the incident field. Among all the theoretical techniques used to study bioelectromagnetism is the numeric 'Finite difference time domain' (FDTD) method which has been widely used.

2.3 Theoretical model for ELF

At a macroscopic level, the interactions of ELF fields with humans and other living organisms can be described in a quantitative and relatively simple manner through the Maxwell's equations.

In the typical human exposure situation, the ELF field is applied through air hence the physical model under study contemplates a grounded or isolated human being and the air in its near environment, such as the case shown in Figure 2.1. At low frequencies, i.e. in the range between 50 Hz and 5 kHz, the wavelength of the EM fields in air varies between 6000 and 60 km. In materials with the electrical and magnetic properties of living tissues, ELF field has a long wavelength, being much bigger than the size of the human body. Consequently, the quasi-static EM field theory is valid and the electric **E** and magnetic **H** fields are decoupled [15]. Figure 2.2 shows the wavelength resulting from a 60-Hz incident field inside different tissues.

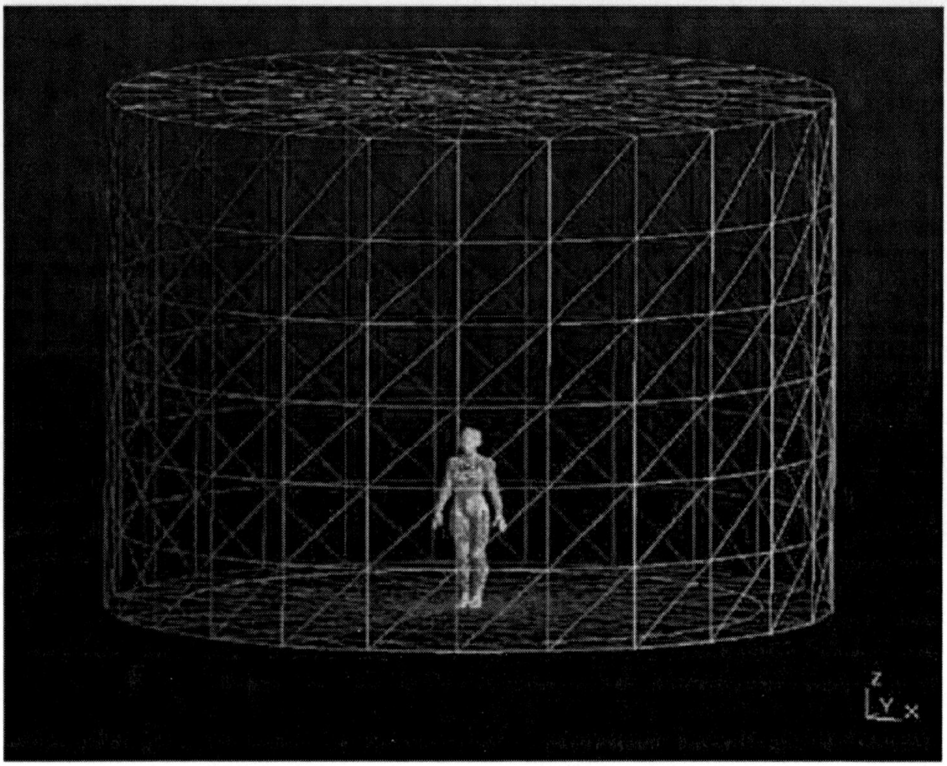

Figure 2.1: Human body conceptual model.

The units used for ELF electric and magnetic fields are defined as the function of the forces they exert on an electric charge q. In case of an ELF electric field with intensity **E**, the force $\mathbf{F}_e$, exerted on a charge at rest is given by Coulomb's law, $\mathbf{F} = q\mathbf{E}$. With **F** in newtons and q in coulombs, the SI unit for the electric field intensity **E** is V/m. An ELF magnetic field with flux density **B** is defined in terms of the force $\mathbf{F}_m$ exerted on a charge moving with velocity v according to Lorentz's law, $\mathbf{F}_m = q(v \times \mathbf{B})$. With **F** in newtons, q in coulombs and v in m/s, the SI unit for the magnetic flux density **B** is Tesla. The set of Maxwell's equations [51] expressed in a lossy, dielectric medium, such as tissue, are of the form

$$\nabla \cdot \mathbf{E} = \rho/\varepsilon \quad \nabla \cdot \mathbf{B} = 0, \tag{M1}$$

$$\nabla \times \mathbf{E} = -\frac{\partial \mathbf{B}}{\partial t} \quad \nabla \times H = J + \frac{\partial(\varepsilon \mathbf{E})}{\partial t}, \tag{M2}$$

where ∇ denotes the divergence of a vector function $\nabla \times$ its curl, t is the time, ρ is the charge density and $\mathbf{J}$ represents the conduction currents. The magnetic field $\mathbf{H}$ is related to the magnetic flux density $\mathbf{B}$ by the permeability μ, i.e. $\mathbf{B} = \mu\mathbf{H}$ and the electric field $\mathbf{E}$ is related with the electric displacement by the permittivity ε, $\mathbf{D} = \varepsilon\mathbf{E}$.

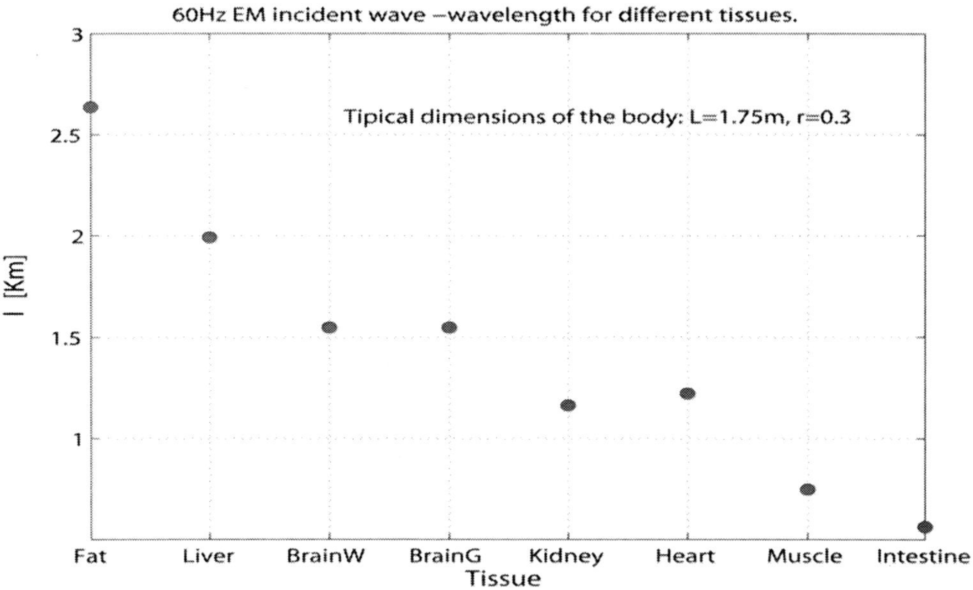

Figure 2.2: Wavelength in different tissues for an incident 60-Hz EM field [50].

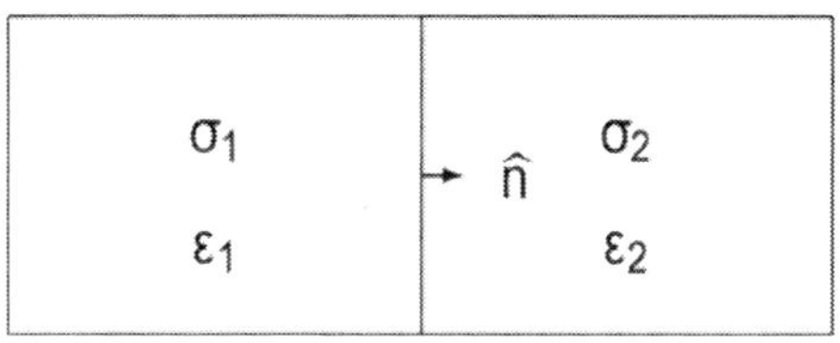

Figure 2.3: Interface between two regions of different properties.

Assuming that the fields are harmonic, they can be represented as [51]

$$\mathbf{E}(r,t) = \mathbf{E}(r)\, e^{-j\omega t}, \tag{2.1}$$

where $j^2 = -1$, $\mathbf{E}(r)$ is in general complex with a magnitude and a phase that change with position, ω is the angular frequency of the incident field and t is the time.

Taking into account that $\partial\mathbf{D}/\partial t = -j\omega e^{j\omega t}\mathbf{D}$ Maxwell's equations become a set of equations of the complex magnitudes which only depend on the position r:

$$\nabla \cdot \mathbf{E} = \rho/\varepsilon \quad \nabla \cdot \mathbf{H} = 0, \tag{M1'}$$

$$\nabla \times \mathbf{E} = -j\mu\omega\mathbf{H} \quad \nabla \times \mathbf{H} = J + j\omega\varepsilon\mathbf{E}. \tag{M2'}$$

When considering the human exposure to high voltage and low intensities systems, such as transmission lines, the most influential field is the electric one and displacement currents can be neglected. The displacement currents are represented by the term $\partial\mathbf{B}/\partial t$ [51].

In this way, the second term in the first equation (M2') vanishes, i.e. $\partial\mathbf{B}/\partial t = -j\mu\omega\mathbf{H} << \nabla\times\mathbf{E}$. Therefore, at these frequencies and in the case of high-voltage low-intensity exposure $\nabla\times\mathbf{E}\sim 0$. Consequently, **E** can be represented by the gradient of the complex scalar potential field φ. In this scope, the electrostatic formulation remains valid ($\nabla\times\mathbf{E}\sim 0$).

$$\mathbf{E} = -\nabla\varphi. \tag{2.2}$$

Making use of the constitutive relation which relate the conductive current **J** to the electric field **E** by the conductivity σ,

$$\mathbf{J} = \sigma\mathbf{E}. \tag{2.3}$$

So, directly from equation (M2'), expressing **E** as a function of φ and applying the constitutive relations, the following expression for the electric scalar potential is obtained:

$$\nabla\cdot[(\sigma + j\omega\varepsilon)\nabla\varphi] = 0. \tag{2.4}$$

Therefore, for ELF, equation (2.4) is the governing equation for the air and the tissues.

The conduction currents are represented by the term $\sigma\mathbf{E}$, while the displacement currents are represented by the term $\omega\varepsilon\mathbf{E}$. Then, the ratio between the conduction currents and the displacement current is characterised by the value of $\omega\varepsilon/\sigma$.

At ELF frequencies, tissue conductivities are of the order of 0.2 S/m and electric permittivity 10^{-10} F/m. Hence, for a 60-Hz incident field, $\omega = 377\ \mathrm{s}^{-1}$, the ratio $\omega\varepsilon/\sigma$ is of the order of 3.77×10^{-10}. Thus, the biological tissue behaves as a good conductor and its permittivity does not intervene in the calculations.

The air is assumed to be a perfect dielectric with null conductivity and permittivity $\varepsilon_0 = 8.85\times10^{-12}$ F/m.

2.3.1 Interface matching conditions

When considering the human exposure problem, the air is modelled as a medium in contact with the skin of the human body, which represents the interface between the two media. While in the interior of the human body, tissues can be modelled as volumes with different material properties and their surfaces represent the interface between different media. The conductivity (σ) and permittivity (ε) are both considered constant within each sub-domain of the body or the air. Figure 2.3 shows the interface between two regions (1 and 2) of different properties. The unit vector $\hat{n}$ is the normal of the surface dividing the two media.

The conservation of the normal component of the electric field across the interface [51] is expressed in the following equation:

$$[\mathbf{E}\cdot\hat{\mathrm{n}}]_{(1)} - [\mathbf{E}\cdot\hat{\mathrm{n}}]_{(2)} = 0, \tag{2.5}$$

where superscripts '1' and '2' indicate the two media.

In terms of the electric potential the previous relation leads to the following condition:

$$\left[(\sigma + j\omega\varepsilon)\frac{\partial\varphi}{\partial n}\right]_{(1)} = \left[(\sigma + j\omega\varepsilon)\frac{\partial\varphi}{\partial n}\right]_{(2)}. \tag{2.6}$$

In general, φ is regarded as a complex potential $\varphi = \varphi R + j\varphi I$. Then equation (2.6) can be split into two equations. When the interface between the air and biological tissue is considered, medium (1) = (AIR) and medium (2) = (BIO).

As stated before, at ELF, conducting properties are dominant, i.e. $\sigma_{(\mathrm{BIO})} >> \omega\varepsilon_{(\mathrm{BIO})}$ for the different biological tissues. Under the previous assumptions, equation (2.6) can be decoupled as presented below. First, it is possible to assign any arbitrary value for the phase of the potential in one of the media. Therefore, for the incident field, $[\varphi I]_{(\mathrm{AIR})}$ can be equal to zero provided that the field in the air has no space dependent phase, thus resulting in the following expression for the interface between air and biological tissue:

$$\begin{aligned} \left[\sigma\frac{\partial\varphi_R}{\partial n}\right]_{(\mathrm{BIO})} &= 0, \\ \left[\sigma\frac{\partial\varphi_I}{\partial n}\right]_{(\mathrm{BIO})} &= \left[\omega\varepsilon\frac{\partial\varphi_R}{\partial n}\right]_{(\mathrm{AIR})}. \end{aligned} \tag{2.7}$$

On the other hand, for interfaces mediating the two regions of biological tissue $_{(\mathrm{BIO1})}$ and $_{(\mathrm{BIO2})}$, the following relations can be derived:

$$\left[\sigma\frac{\partial\varphi_R}{\partial n}\right]_{(\mathrm{BIO1})} = \left[\sigma\frac{\partial\varphi_R}{\partial n}\right]_{(\mathrm{BIO2})}, \tag{2.8}$$

$$\left[\sigma\frac{\partial\varphi_I}{\partial n}\right]_{(\mathrm{BIO1})} = \left[\sigma\frac{\partial\varphi_I}{\partial n}\right]_{(\mathrm{BIO2})}. \tag{2.9}$$

Considering that $\partial\varphi/\partial n = \mathbf{E}_n$, the boundary condition between air and the surface of the body, represented by equation (2.7), relates the intensity of the normal electric field inside the body $\mathbf{E}_n^{(\mathrm{BIO})}$ and in the air $\mathbf{E}_n^{(\mathrm{AIR})}$. Therefore, the value of the normal field at the interface for the biological tissue can be estimated by

$$\mathbf{E}_n^{(\mathrm{BIO})} = \frac{\omega\varepsilon_0}{\sigma^{(\mathrm{BIO})}}\mathbf{E}_n^{(\mathrm{AIR})}. \tag{2.10}$$

Although tissue conductivities vary depending on the particular tissue, a typical value of conductivity that represents biological tissues at ELF is 0.2 S/m, hence for a 60-Hz incident electric field, the internal field in the surface of the body is estimated by $\mathbf{E}_n^{(\mathrm{BIO})} \approx 2\times10^{-8}\mathbf{E}_n^{(\mathrm{AIR})}$.

2.4 Different sources of exposure at ELF

Due to the uncoupling of the electromagnetic field at ELF, the exposure can be analysed separately. The highest level of exposure to ELF electric fields occurs under high-voltage transmission lines and in substations, where the ambient field levels can reach intensities of 15–20 kV/m. In contrast, the highest levels of ELF magnetic field exposure occur in the home or work-place. Depending on the purpose of the substation, they generally produce a magnetic field of up to 2 μT close to them and fall rapidly with distance.

Table 2.4 shows levels of 60-Hz electric and magnetic field that are frequently encountered under distribution and high-voltage transmission lines in substations and in homes due to normal appliances.

Figure 2.4 shows a 275-kV power transmission line passing over a neighbourhood in Southampton, UK.

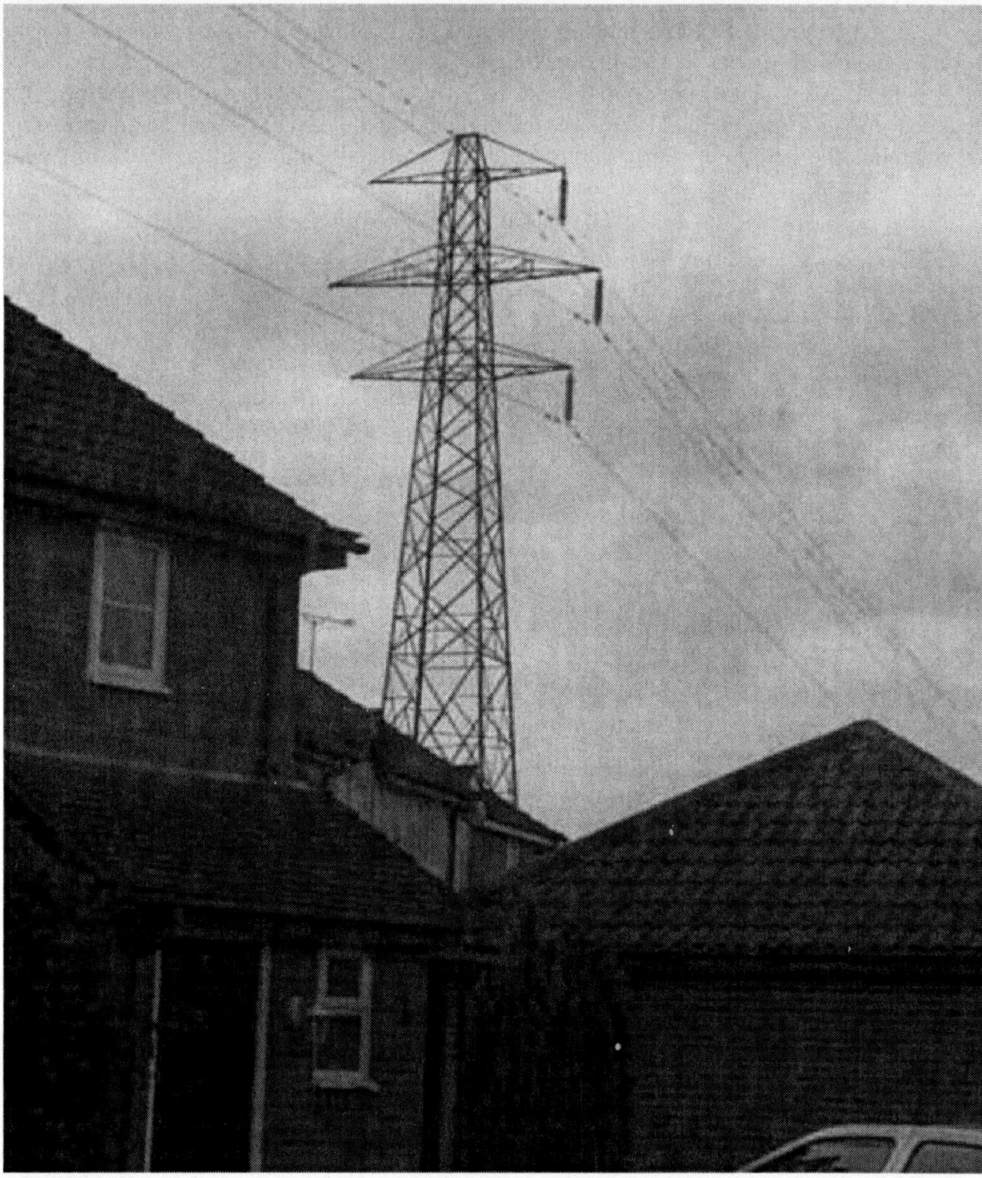

Figure 2.4: 275-kV power transmission line across an urban area. Totton, Southampton, UK.

Table 2.4: Typical levels of **E** and **H** in UK power lines, substations and homes [**E**] = V/m and [**H**] = μT [56].

Typical UK lines	400 and 275 kV	132 kV	33 and 11 kV
E_{max} (under line)	11,000	4000	700
E_{typ} (under line)	4000	1000–2000	200
E_{typ} (25 m to side)	200–500	100–200	10–20
B_{max} (under line)	100	40	7
B_{typ} (under line)	5–10	0.5–2	0.2–0.5
B_{typ} (25 m to side)	1–2	0.05–0.2	0.01–0.05
Substations	Outside	Indoors	
H	0.1		
E	≈0		
Home appliances	H close	H 1 m away	
Electric razor	2000	0.3	
Vacuum cleaner	800	2	
TV	50	0.2	
Washing machine	50	0.2	
Bedside clock	50	0.02	
Fridge	2	0.0	

2.5 Summary

This chapter presents an introduction to the human body exposure to ELF electromagnetic fields.

A general classification of the EM radiation according to its frequency, type of interaction with the biological tissues and consequent effects is introduced together with a differentiation between non-thermal and thermal effects.

Dosimetry parameters and possible harmful effects at different frequencies are sketched. The theoretical basis for the EM modelling of the problem of a human body exposed to an ELF field is presented. Departing from the macroscopic Maxwell equations for imperfect conductor material, the governing equations for ELF are derived. This formulation is restricted in frequency by the condition $\omega\varepsilon/\sigma \ll 1$, i.e. up to a few kilo hertz where electric fields and induced currents can be deduced from the solution of potential problems based on Laplace equation.

Proper interface matching conditions between regions of different electrical properties including air-body are provided. Finally, different sources of exposure to ELF fields and the typical levels of electric and magnetic fields that are frequently encountered under high-voltage distribution and transmission lines, near substations and in homes in UK are enumerated.

3

Dielectric properties of biological tissues

3.1 Introduction

Not only for protection from exposure to EM fields but also for its relevance in medical research, it is essential to fully understand the interaction of EM radiation with biological systems as well as the intrinsic EM behaviour of biological matter.

To establish mechanisms of interaction, it is necessary to characterise the electromagnetic properties of biological systems. In order to set the level of approximation, in which study of the problem of EM interaction with living systems is carried out, and choose the correspondent assumptions that yields acceptable results, it is necessary to have a deep understanding of the complex and extremely heterogeneous system represented by biological matter.

This chapter is devoted to the study of the dielectric properties of tissue, summarising the findings that have been studied by authors and references. Schwan made a monumental work on the study of dielectric properties of tissues [57–59] (Foster and Schwan [60], Foster [61], Peters et al. [62], Miklavcic et al. [63], Pavlin et al. [64] at cellular level, Stuchly and Stuchly [65] and Gabriel et al. [66, 67] among others).

Section 3.2 describes the different levels of scales that can be used to model biological tissues. Section 3.3 enumerates the different sources of dielectric measures available in literature and describes the difficulties that arise when performing dielectric parameters measurements. Section 3.4 describes the basis of the interaction between electric field and biological matter and its dependence on frequency.

Particular characteristics of different groups of tissues are analysed in Section 3.5. Section 3.6 focuses on the dielectric properties of tissues at ELF, revising the data available and pointing out differences between measurements. Also, the conduction and displacement currents for some tissues are compared at these frequencies, showing that for most of the tissues the conduction currents are at least one order of magnitude bigger than the displacement currents, allowing in this way to consider only tissue conductivity and to neglect tissue permittivity in the calculations. In Section 3.6.3, a method for estimating tissue conductivity at ELF frequency is outlined. Finally, Sections 3.6.4 and 3.6.5 describe the dielectric data available in the case of pregnant woman and foetus, respectively, and applied the method previously described to estimate tissue conductivity for the pregnant woman and foetus.

3.2 Modelling biological systems

When dealing with human body, modelling the major difficulties appearing are related to the material properties, as well as to geometrical aspects. The human body or a part of it is a very complex system made up of many sub-domains with different properties which may interact with one another [1]. In this way, the number of variables necessary to define a model could lead to a very high number of unknowns. Another problem to deal with is the modelling and accurate description of the sources that generate the EM fields. In general, in a real situation these sources are time dependant and may vary in location, intensity, frequency and duration. Additionally, the human body also may move, changing not only the geometry definition of the problem but also the material properties may be modified. Regarding the material properties, the first problem is that they have to be identified and their properties have to be defined. Once identified, there is still the problem that these properties also depend on the activity of the person and vary with the environment, the age of the person [68] and in some degree even the sex. Furthermore, the proportion of each tissue varies from one subject to another which makes the representation of one single model not representative. Moreover, the orders of magnitude for the properties of different tissues differ largely from each other, which can introduce not only numerical difficulties but also changes in the applied physical approximations [1].

3.2.1 The scale

In order to study and model a biological system in particular, the description has to be performed in a particular scale. While from a macroscopic point of view the human body can be considered as a whole, made up of several homogeneous tissues, organs and fluids; from a microscopic view each tissue is made up of cells that perform similar functions.

On a microscopic scale, human tissue is a very complex structure. Roughly speaking, it consists of cells suspended in aqueous conducting medium. In this way a tissue has to be considered as an inhomogeneous suspension of particles in a solvent, leading to a two domain representation: extracellular and intracellular media [62]. The microscopic representation is complicated by the variety of cell shapes and their distribution inside the tissue as well as by the different properties of the extracellular media. Regarding the cell shapes, although spheres, spheroids and ellipsoids may be reasonable models for suspended cells, the geometry of the cells in tissues is very irregular. Furthermore, in a tissue every cell differs in its shape from the rest [64].

From a macroscopic point of view, tissue can be considered as a homogeneous volume and its material properties can be treated as 'effective' quantities pro-mediated over the whole volume [62]. In this way, the human body is regarded as a piece-wise homogeneous volume in which each tissue is described by a different effective quantity. Generally, different tissues have physical properties that may differ largely from one another. For instance, there are electrically active tissues such as nerves, muscles, tissue of the brain and heart. Electric or magnetic fields may excite these tissues by several mechanisms, generating currents flowing inside the body. Even the endogenous biological currents that naturally flow inside the body are capable of generating EM fields sufficiently large to be measured outside of the body by using, for example, electro- and magneto-encephalography (EEG-MEG) in the case of the brain, or electro-magneto-cardiography (ECG-MCG) in case of the heart [63]. Moreover, there are some tissues like fat or bone that are electrically more passive.

In order to represent a biological system, intermediate scales can also be considered, due to the special characteristics of some tissues, which have stratified organisation. For instance, in the case of the skin, the tissue is composed of three layers, namely epidermis, dermis and a fat layer. Although each layer has different material properties, it is possible to consider an effective parameter for the composite material [63].

3.2.2 Coupling different scales problems

The previous arguments and considerations lead to the necessity to analyse the interaction between external EM fields and biological systems at different levels, and to integrate the macroscopic and microscopic scales [61]. Firstly, the coupling between external fields and the different homogeneous volumes inside the body has to be considered (macrodosimetry). Secondly, as a result of the fields induced in different volume conductors within the body, induced fields at cellular or sub-cellular level arise (microdosimetry). And finally, it is necessary to determine the biological response, if exists, to the local field [61].

3.3 Available data on dielectric properties

Dielectric properties of biological tissues have been extensively studied theoretically and experimentally. Early works of Cook has been performed in 1951 [69, 70]. An extremely large contribution is made by Schwan (1957) and his colleges who dominated the literature in the 1950s and 1960s [58]. Durney has reviewed and tabulated his previous work in 1986 [50]. Schwan and Foster in 1980 [59] and Foster and Schwan (1989) [60], critically reviewed electrical properties of tissues from DC to 20 GHz. They studied the principles behind dielectric relaxation, analysed the difference between dielectric properties of normal and cancerous tissues and summarised advances in counter ion polarisation theories. They studied the correlation between water content of a tissue and its dielectric properties, stabilising the empirical correlations with tissue water content. In addition, they presented a comprehensive table of dielectric properties for different tissues. Stuchly and Stuchly in 1980 [65] tabulated the dielectric properties in the frequency range from 10 kHz to 10 GHz. In 1990, Duck extended this survey. Gabriel et al. in 1996 made a very extensive and detailed literature survey and extracted the dielectric properties of tissues (of the previous five) decades in the frequency range from 10 Hz to 20 GHz, presenting them in a graphical format [66]. They also included their own measurements of the dielectric properties for more than 30 animal and human excised and in vivo tissue type over a wide frequency range [71], and finally presented a parametric empirical model to predict the variation of dielectric properties of tissues as a function of frequency [67].

3.3.1 Measurements

Despite the fact that the material properties have been extensively studied, the effective conductivity and permittivity for the various tissues are not accurately known. In particular, for ELF range, below 100 Hz, data in the literature on specific conductivity and relative permittivity for most tissues is very scarce, do not exist at all or show wide variations [71]. The reason is because for this frequency range experimental errors can ruin the measurements. On the other hand, measurements are complicated by several factors [62, 71].

1. Inhomogeniety**.** In fact, tissue is a very inhomogeneous material. Not only the cells itself are inhomogeneous but tissues are comprised of different types of cell, with different sizes and functions as well. For instance, bone contains osteoblasts, osteocytes and osteoclasts embedded in a collagen matrix as well as bone marrow with stroma cells [72]. The tissue is perfused with blood and linked to the central nervous system by neurons. Consequently, it

is difficult to extrapolate from the dielectric properties of a cell suspension to those of a whole tissue.

2. Non-linearity. In order not to trigger a response, the currents applied have to be low, thus they are only representative for linear responses, i.e. responses for large field intensities can have different material properties.
3. Anisotropy. Some tissues, such as bone and skeletal muscle, are anisotropic [73]. Therefore, it is necessary to establish the direction in which the EF is applied in relation to the major axis of the tissues, i.e. longitudinal or transversal. Skeletal muscle is probably the best example of this variation, in which the conductivity can be up to 10 times lower along the length of the muscle fibres compared to the perpendicular orientation.
4. Condition of the tissue. For measurements taken place in vitro, the accuracy may be low because tissue properties change rapidly when they are taken outside from the body [74]. In general, the conductivity increases with time of excise. On the contrary, if the measurements are carried out in vivo, commonly animal tissues are used instead of human tissue. It is not clear, however, whether animal tissues have the same material properties as human tissue. Additionally, the major problem in this case is that the measurements also are affected by the tissues in the surroundings.
5. Electrode polarisation. There are intrinsic errors related to the measurement itself. Two main sources of systematic errors are electrode polarisation and lead inductance, due to a large capacitance and resistance at the interface between electrode and tissue, particularly at low frequencies ranges [71].
6. Gabriel applied a correction to the effect of electrode polarisation, but still considered the possibility that the dielectric parameters they tabulated below 1 kHz might be under-corrected and that this source of errors might affect the dielectric parameters by up to a factor of two or three. However, because tissue impedance at low frequencies is almost entirely resistive, permittivity errors do not play any major role.

For all the exposed reasons, considerable caution must be taken in the interpretation of electrical measurements.

3.4 Theoretical aspects. Biological matter in electric field

Characterisation of the material properties of biological tissues at macroscopic level has to be performed by reference to the microscopic structure of tissue, since macroscopic properties and behaviour of biological tissues are closely related to the properties and behaviour of their constitutive cells.

3.4.1 Definition of the dielectric properties

At macroscopic level, the interaction of EM fields and biological tissues can be described by the Maxwell equations [51] as described in Chapter 2, Section 2.3. As human tissues are non-magnetic materials, the permeability μ of the entire body is almost equal to the permeability of the vacuum μ_o.

In order to characterise biological tissue's electric properties, it is useful to start considering the electrical properties of simpler materials, which in general can be broadly separated into to two types of materials: conductors and insulators [51]. Although this analysis does not consider the complexity of biological tissues, it yields some illuminating insight on the phenomena involved with the dielectric character of biological materials. In a conductor, the electric charges move freely in response to an applied EM field, whereas in an insulator the charges are fixed and not able to move.

If a conductor is placed in an electric field, due to polarisation phenomenon, charges move to the surface in response to the field and the electric field inside the material vanishes. In the case of an insulator or perfect dielectric, there are no free charges but if the material is polar, the dipoles respond to an applied electric field $\mathbf{E}_a$ by reorienting themselves, generating an $\mathbf{E}_p$ field, which opposes the applied field. If it is a non-polar material, its molecules will be polarised in response to the field, generating as well an $\mathbf{E}_p$ field opposite to the applied field [51]. The net field inside the material will be the resultant of both fields as follows:

$$\mathbf{E}_{\text{net}} = \mathbf{E}_{\text{a}} + \mathbf{E}_{\text{p}}. \tag{3.1}$$

If the material is a conductor, all the free charges will move to its surface, hence the field generated in response to the external field is such that equals the applied field, leading to a net zero field inside the material.

If the net field inside the material does not vanish, it will be reduced by an amount that depends on the ability of the material to transport charges. This reduction is characterised by the dielectric constant or relative permittivity [51] according to the following equation:

$$\mathbf{E}_{\text{net}} = \frac{\mathbf{E}_{\text{a}}}{\varepsilon_{\text{r}}}. \tag{3.2}$$

The dielectric constant ε_r expresses the relation between the permittivity ε of a medium and the permittivity of vacuum ε_o [51], i.e.

$$\varepsilon_{\text{r}} = \frac{\varepsilon}{\varepsilon_{\text{o}}}. \tag{3.3}$$

In general, biological tissues exhibit characteristics of conductors and insulators at the same time [50] as they are made of polar molecules, such as water, but they also have charges that can move in a restricted way. In biological tissues, charge carriers are ions. In this way, biological tissue behaves as an electrolytic conductor in which ions are able to migrate in response to an external applied field. But at the same time, they exhibit the characteristics of dielectric materials such as polarisation and orientation of permanent dipoles with the external applied field [60].

Biological tissues are heterogeneous and complex in their microscopic structure; charges can be trapped at interfaces, reducing the amount of charge that may be transported [50]. At the same time, as the ions can be positive and negative, if they are trapped, this yield to an effective internal polarisation acting like a large dipole. Hence, the different mechanisms of polarisation lead to a frequency dependency of the tissue properties and to several dielectric dispersions [50, 60].

Assuming that tissues are macroscopically homogeneous, as described in Chapter 2, the electrical properties of tissues can be described by two parameters, namely the permittivity ε and the conductivity σ.

Considering tissue to be homogeneous at macroscopic level is supported experimentally since the conductivity and the permittivity are parameters that can be measured for different types of tissues [62].

Whereas the conductivity characterises the material ability to transport charge throughout the material by response to an applied electric field, the permittivity characterises its tendency either to store charge or to polarise. As a result, a perfect dielectric is a material that has no conductivity, whereas a perfect conductor has no permittivity. Table 3.1 illustrates the typical variations on the conductivity for common materials.

Table 3.1: Conductivities for common materials.

Type of material	Typical conductivities σ [S/m]
Perfect conductor	∞
Metals	10^4
Electrolytes	$1–10^2$
Bio-tissues	$10^{-4}–10^2$
Semiconductors	$10^{-4}–1$
Dielectrics	10^{-10}
Perfect dielectric	0

Conductivity values for common dielectrics are very low, lower than 10^{-10} S/m, whereas for metals the conductivity values are high, higher than 10^4 S/m. Between metals and insulators are semiconductors with conductivity in the range of $1–10^{-4}$ S/m and electrolytes in which conduction occurs by transport of ions in solution with conductivity values of the order of $1–10^2$ S/m. Tissue can be considered as a collection of electrolytes contained within membranes. Therefore, the complexity of its composition at microscopic level yields spread conductivity and permittivity values.

Making use of the constitutive relations [51], the conduction current resulting by the transport of charges is given by

$$\mathbf{J}_c = \sigma\mathbf{E}. \tag{3.4}$$

In this way, in the second term of equation (M2') from Chapter 2is as follows:

$$\nabla \times \mathbf{H} = \mathbf{J} + i\omega\varepsilon\mathbf{E}, \tag{M2'}$$

Where the sources of **H** can be expressed as an addition of conductive currents given by the first term and displacement currents represented by the second term as follows:

$$\mathbf{J}_d = -i\omega\varepsilon\mathbf{E}. \tag{3.5}$$

Hence, the total current density $\mathbf{J}_{tot}$ flowing in a material is given by the conduction current plus the displacement current by the following expression:

$$\mathbf{J}_{tot} = \mathbf{J}_c + \mathbf{J}_d = (\sigma - i\omega\varepsilon)\mathbf{E} = -i\omega\varepsilon^*\mathbf{E}. \tag{3.6}$$

where ω is the frequency of the applied field and ε^* is known as the complex permittivity and defined in this formalism as $\varepsilon^* = \varepsilon - i(\sigma/\omega)$.

If the conductivity σ and the permittivity ε do not depend on the frequency, it follows from equations (3.4) and (3.5) that the conduction current is constant, whereas the displacement current increases with frequency. Consequently, at low frequencies the material will behave as a conductor and in a constant field the displacement current will be zero. In contrast, at higher frequencies induced currents will become more important.

However, for biological tissues, the material properties vary with the frequency of the applied field. These variations are called dispersions [50]. Dispersions can be explained in terms of the polarisation and the motion of the charge carriers. At low frequency, the dipoles reorient by the action of an applied field, while the charge carriers are travelling through the material in one direction during a period of time. During this travel, they may reach to a charged interface in which they may be trapped [63]. Hence, the conduction of charges will decrease. Therefore, at low frequencies, the permittivity will be high and the conductivity low.

As the frequency increases, it is more difficult for the dipoles to follow the changes in the external field, hence the polarisation decreases. Instead, for the charge carriers, they travel shorter distances before they change their direction, resulting in the decrease of the possibility of being trapped by an interface. Consequently, the conductivity will increase and the permittivity will decrease [63].

3.4.2 Dispersions

In real biological tissue, the variation of the material properties with the frequency of the applied field, i.e. dispersions, may be more or less important depending on the particular tissue [50].

Figure 3.1 represents a schematic view for the variation of the real part of the relative permittivity for a wide frequency range. It decreases in distinct steps as the frequency increases. A dispersion will then be the transition from one level to another [50]. For frequencies below 100 Hz, there is a level in which the relative permittivity reaches approximately 10^7–10^8 and then decreases as the frequency increases to 10 kHz into a second level of 10^5. Between 100 Hz and 100 kHz, most tissues, with the exception of the anisotropic tissues, show almost no frequency dependence. After some slow decrease from 100 MHz to some GHz, reaches a third level of about 80. This last value is that of the dielectric constant of water at microwaves. Schwan [58] was the first who observed the three levels and major dispersions in which the properties of biological tissue are characterised. He named them as α, β and γ dispersions, respectively. Evidently, different mechanisms account for low frequency, radio frequency and microwave frequency.

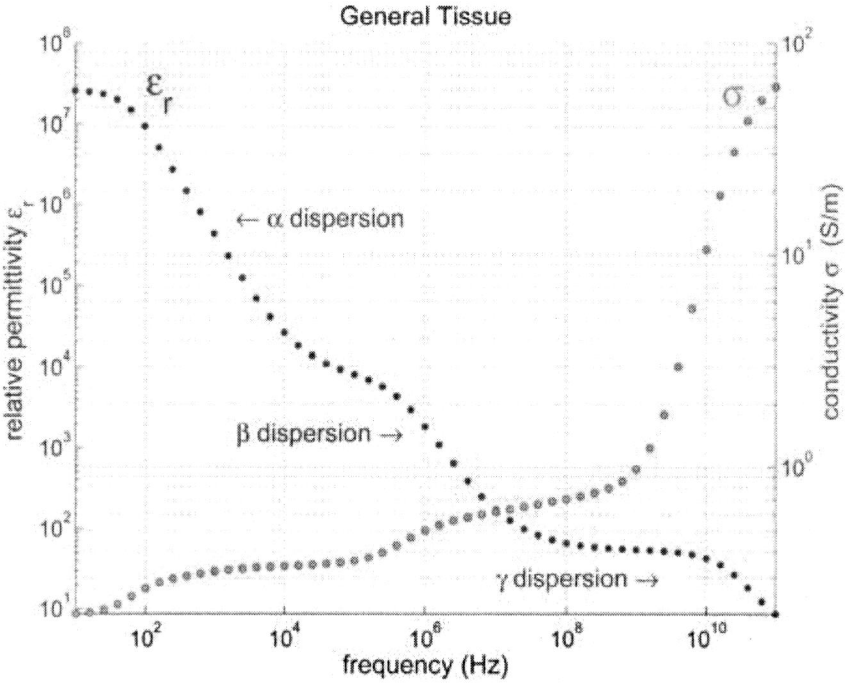

Figure 3.1: Idealised frequency dependence of the complex permittivity and conductivity of a soft tissue.

In an attempt to reproduce the measured behaviour of dispersive materials, two approaches have been used to model them: from a macroscopic view, the behaviour of the system can be reproduced by circuit models which consider capacitor and resistors. On the contrary, from a microscopic view, the system is analysed considering its constituents: cells, fluid in which the cells are immersed and ions.

- Macroscale behaviour. Debye model uses a parallel RC element which is able to reproduce one dispersion. Cole and Cole (1941) [75] performed a more complex model of resistors and capacitors that has been applied very successfully to a wide variety of materials over the last 60 years. The complexity of the dispersions illustrated in Figure 3.1 has been reproduced by Gabriel et al. [67] by a four successive Cole–Cole dispersion model which can be explicitly written in terms of the parameters that have been tabulated in their work for the 30 tissues types along the four regions of dispersions.
- Cellular level scale behaviour. At these scale the biological tissue can be represented as two different phases basically; extracellular fluid and intracellular space. The dispersions result from the interaction of the applied field with the constituents of the biological tissue at cellular and molecular level. The cell consists of a conductive interior and a very poor conductive membrane. However, this membrane has pores and gap junctions by which, under certain conditions, it can communicate with the extracellular fluid or another cells.

  At low frequencies, tissue can be regarded simply as a suspension of non-conductive particles in a conducting fluid, as the cell membrane being of the order of 10^{-5} less conductive than the intracellular media and provides the insulation.

  At frequencies in the MHz range, capacitive coupling across this membrane becomes more important. Beginning in this range, the dispersive properties of the membrane and ultimately the intra-cellular space must also be considered. The main characteristics can be briefly explained as follows [66].

  The extremely high values of permittivity for the first level reflect the fact that the charges are trapped in the internal interfaces surrounding the cell membrane and forming a counter-ion cloud. Thus, they are not related to dipole orientation. In fact, even at the lowest frequency a residual or DC conductivity σ_o exists (σ is not zero), as it can be seen from Figure 3.1.
- The low-frequency α dispersion is associated with the counter-ion polarisation along cell membranes as well as ionic diffusion processes at the cellular membrane.
- The β dispersion, in the hundred of kHz region is caused mainly by the polarisation of cellular membranes which act as barriers to the flow of ions between the intra- and extra-cellular media. Other contributions to the β dispersion come from the polarisation of proteins and other organic macromolecules.
- The γ dispersion, in the GHz region, is due to polarisation of water molecules.

3.5 General dielectric properties of some tissues

Dielectric properties differ largely depending on the considered tissue. In Figures 3.2 and 3.3, the conductivity and relative permittivity for fat, muscle and body fluid is presented for a wide frequency range. Data has been obtained using the parameterised relation proposed by Gabriel et al. (1996c) [67]. With the exception of the anisotropic tissues, for frequencies below 100 kHz, tissues with high proportion of water, like body fluid, show almost no frequency dependence. In particular, the proportion of water or fluid present in the considered tissue has a significant role in the consequent behaviour and dielectric properties of tissue. According to a recent study [76] of electrical resistivity of human tissues in the frequency range from 100 Hz to 10 MHz, a relation was found between the resistivity and the water content of some tissues. The low water content of bone and fat explains their lower conductivities, while the high water content of other tissues explains their high conductivity. Besides, the anisotropic structures of biological tissues may also contribute significantly to the measured electrical properties. Consequently, tissues having similar behaviour can be grouped as follows according to their water content.

- Blood and brain have high water content and conduct electric current relatively well.
- Lungs, skin, fat and bone are relatively poor conductors.
- Liver, spleen and muscles are intermediate in their conductivities.

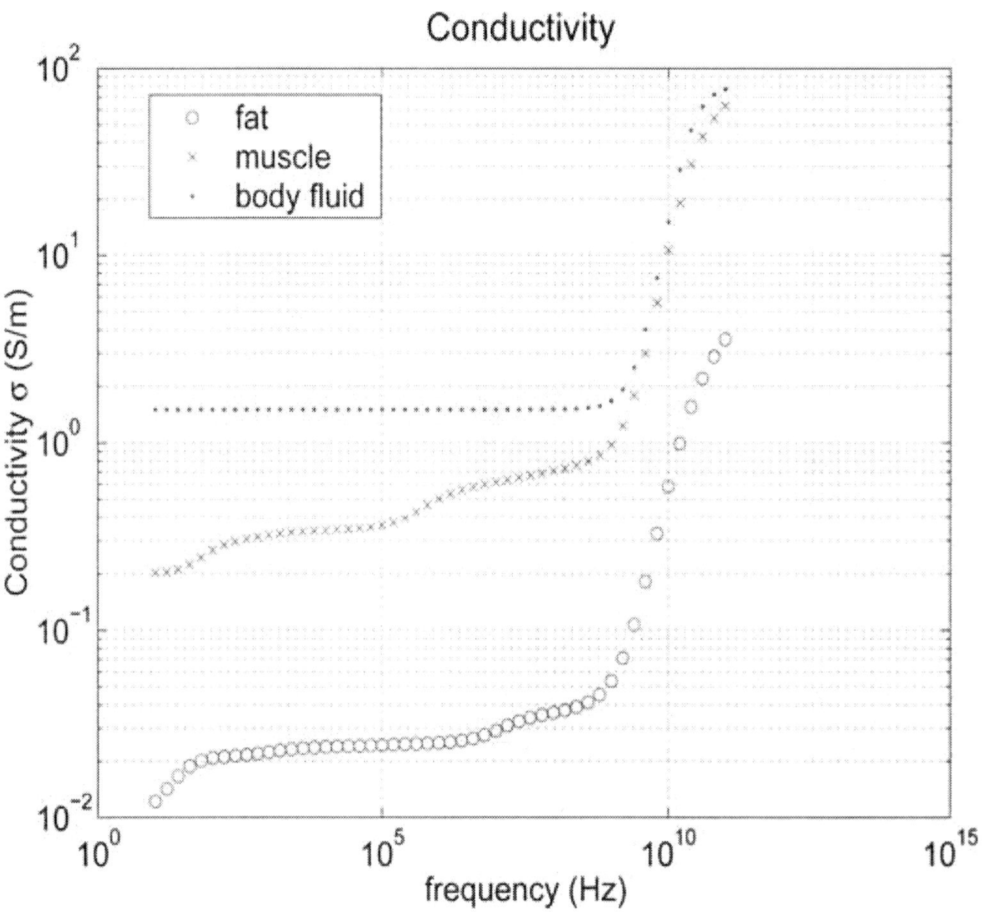

Figure 3.2: Conductivity and permittivity for a soft tissue, a wet tissue and a fluid tissue for a wide frequency range.

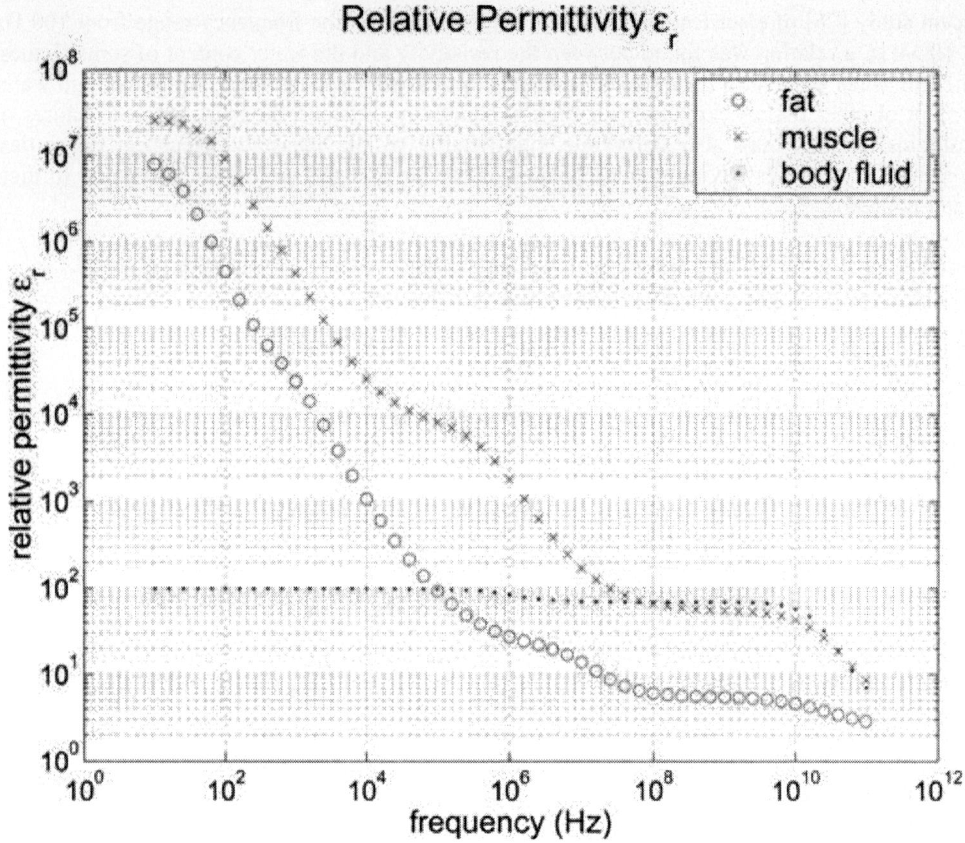

Figure 3.3: Permittivity for a soft tissue, a wet tissue and a fluid tissue for a wide frequency range.

3.6 Biological tissue at ELF

After the previous considerations, data extracted in order to carry out the studies described in this book is presented in the following paragraphs.

At ELF frequencies the data available is scarce, and the conditions and biomaterials in which the experiments have been carried out are very dissimilar; ranging from human samples to animals ones, such as rats, bovines and canine samples, experiments performed at different temperatures and with different techniques and with samples taken either in vivo or in vitro. Table 3.2 above shows the data ranges of the conductivities and relative permittivities of some tissues at 100 Hz. The data has been extracted from measurements reported in references [66, 71]. The data has been selected analysing the results from various studies and choosing the measurements that report the minimum and maximum values of the conductivity and permittivity. The superscript 'a' indicates that the data correspond to the same study. Where there is no superscript, the pair of linked data corresponds to 2 minimum or 2 maximum, respectively. For some particular tissues, such as bone cancellous, white matter or kidney, only one study has been found, thus a unique value is reported in the table. As has been described in the previous sections, the data presented emphasises the wide variations founded in the experimental data available.

Table 3.2: Data Ranges of specific conductivities and relative permittivities of tissues measured at 100 Hz [66, 71].

Tissue type	Measured conductivity [S/m] Min. value	Measured conductivity [S/m] Max. value	Measured relative permittivity Min. value	Measured relative permittivity Max. value
Muscle				
Transversal	0.08	0.45	3.5×10^5	4×10^6
Longitudinal	0.3	0.8	7×10^6	6×10^7
Liver	0.04	0.12	2×10^5	8×10^6
Lung (infl)	0.05[a]	0.1	4.5×10^5	1.5×10^6[a]
Spleen	0.043	0.1[a]	3.6×10^6[a]	4.5×10^7
Skin (dry)	2×10^{-5}	2×10^{-1}	3×10^3	4×10^4
Fat	0.0015	0.03	6×10^4	2×10^5
Bone cortical	0.006	0.0132	4×10^3	
Bone cancellous	0.18		7×10^5	
White matter	0.023		3×10^7	
Kidney	0.1		3×10^6	
Heart	0.1		3×10^5	3×10^6

[a] Data correspond to the same study.

3.6.1 Relative importance of conductive and displacement currents

The relative importance of the permittivity and conductivity in determining the electrical properties of the tissue can be compared by taking the ratio of the conduction and displacements currents as follows:

$$\frac{|\mathrm{j_c}|}{|\mathrm{j_d}|} = \frac{\sigma}{\omega \varepsilon}, \tag{3.7}$$

where $\varepsilon = \varepsilon_r \varepsilon_0$. In the ELF range, this ratio is very big for almost all tissues, even with the high values of the relative permittivity ε_r that are reached. Figure 3.4 illustrates this situation for the data obtained from the work of Gabriel et al. 1996c [67] using the factors and parameterisation proposed by them, which allows to calculate a reasonable estimate for the conductivity and permittivity for different tissue types. Tissues like body fluid, blood and cerebrospinal fluid have ratios of the order of 10^6–10^7 as can be appreciated in Figure 3.4. However, tissues such as bone cortical, prostate, eyes and bladder have ratios ranging between 10^2 and 10^4. In contrast, for tissues like fat, muscle, heart, skin, uterus, cervix, brain and lung, the ratio fall in the region between 1 and 10 as can be seen in Figure 3.5. Only colon falls to a value smaller than 1.

Therefore, for a wide range of tissues the contribution of the capacitive component is of the order of 10% or smaller. Hence, at low frequencies, biological tissues are essentially conductive in nature.

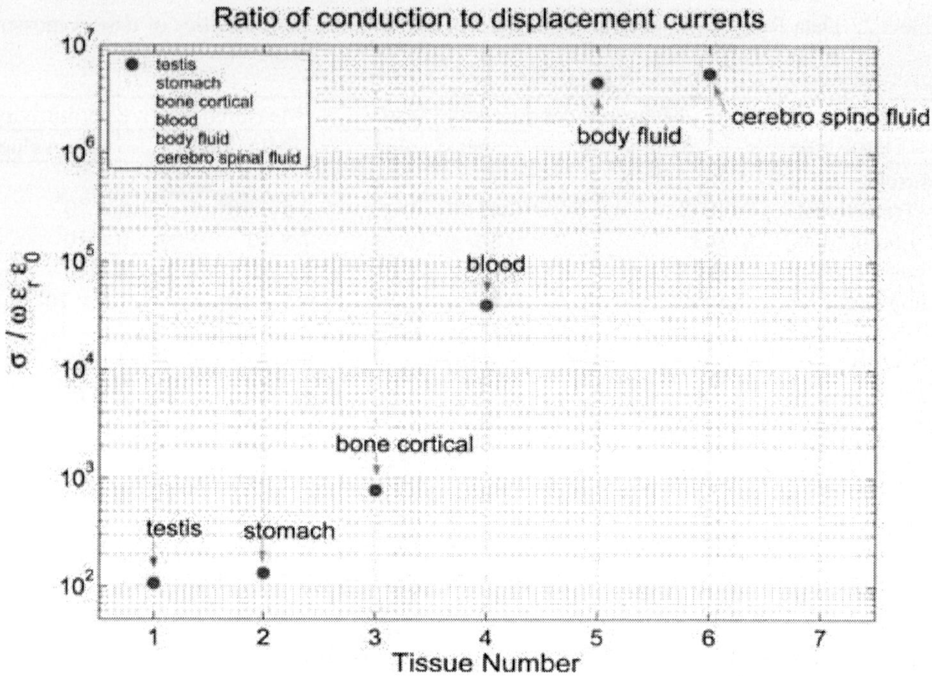

Figure 3.4: Conductive to displacement current ratio in tissues at 60 Hz.

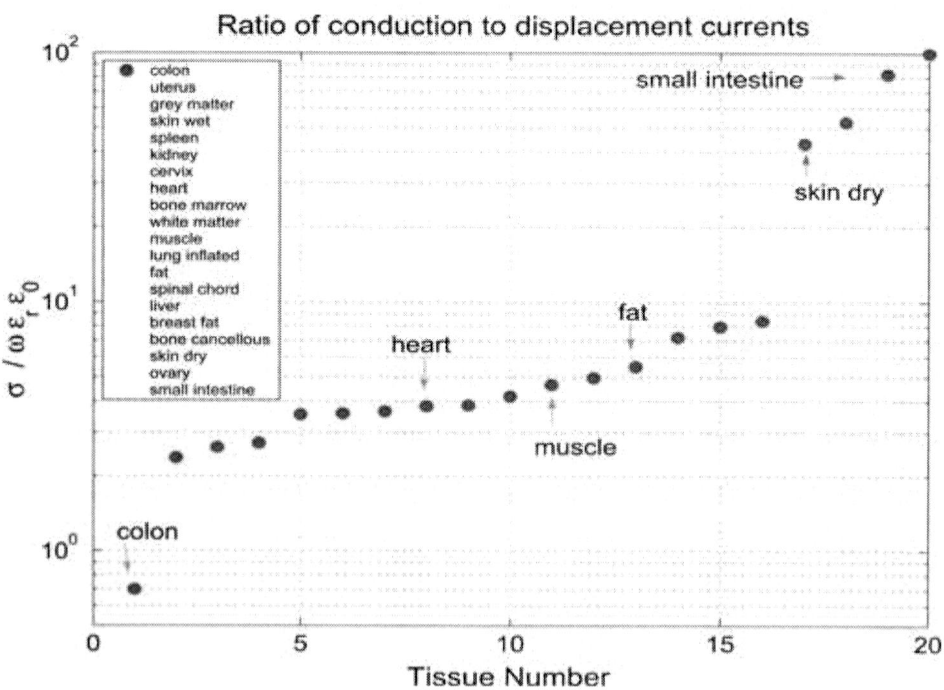

Figure 3.5: Conductive to displacement current ratio in tissues at 60 Hz.

3.6.2 Dielectric data below 100 Hz

On the basis of the fact that below 100 Hz the impedance of biological material is mostly resistive, the contribution of the permittivity will not play a major role and the evaluation of induced current in tissue is based only on conductivity values [71]. In Table 3.3, an estimation for conductivity in S/m of the main body tissues below 100 Hz is presented, extracted from the works of Gabriel et al. (1996). From the parametric relation, the conductivity and the permittivity can be obtained as a function of frequency. These values are the standard set of parameters presently used by most researchers in computational dosimetry. However, Gandhi uses the values tabulated in Table 3.4. Additionally, Faes et al. (1999) [76] conducted a study on electrical resistivity of human tissues in the frequency range from 100 Hz to 10 MHz in order to analyse the large differences that appear between previous studies and measurements. The aim of their work was to investigate systematically the previous findings on resistivities of human tissues in order to obtain an estimate of the real resistivities of various tissues, to quantify the uncertainties of these estimates and to test statistically whether resistivities of tissues differ significantly. Table 3.5 summarises Faes results translated to conductivity values. In their work, it was shown that differences between the mean values of resistivity of most tissues from muscle and internal organs are statistically insignificant. Moreover, as it can be seen in Table 3.5, the reported mean resistivity for skeletal muscle, cardiac muscle, kidney, liver, lung, breast, skin and blood were similar. Only bone, fat and stratum cornea have significant lower conductivities. Based on these results, at these frequencies a model that considers a homogeneous representation for some group of tissues may give a good insight in the evaluation of induced current densities and fields inside the body. In this context, in some studies, it is useful to consider effective values of conductivity integrated along body regions or even the whole body. Table 3.6 summarises the values given by Gabriel for the effective conductivity integrated along the whole body, legs, arms, head, torso and neck. Gabriel et al. has performed the integration of the conductivity of tissue for the values shown in Table 3.3 by allocating the appropriate values to the voxel anatomical human model NORMAN.

Table 3.3: Tissue conductivities at ELF exposures calculated with Gabriel parameterisation formulas [67].

Tissue	Calculated conductivity [S/m]
Bone cortical	0.02
Spinal cord	0.03
Fat	0.04
Breast	0.06
Brain (white matter)	0.06
Bone trabecular	0.07
Liver	0.07
Lung	0.07
Heart muscle	0.08
Kidney	0.09
Spleen	0.09
Brain (grey matter)	0.10
Skin	0.10
Pancreas	0.21
Uterus	0.23

Table 3.3: Tissue conductivities at ELF exposures calculated with Gabriel parameterisation formulas [67]. (*Continued*)

Tissue	Calculated conductivity [S/m]
Vagina	0.23
Eye lens	0.26
Tendons	0.27
Muscle	0.35
Ovaries	0.32
Prostate	0.42
Testis	0.42
Eye Sclera/retina	0.50
Oesophagus	0.52
Stomach	0.52
Thymus	0.52
Thyroid	0.52
Blood	0.70
Intestine small	1.09
Intestine large	1.24
Eye humour	1.50
Duodenum	1.09
Cerebrospinal fluid	2.00
Stomach contents	2.00
Urine	3.30

Table 3.4: Tissue conductivities at ELF exposures used by Gandhi [25].

Tissue	Calculated conductivity [S/m]
Cartilage	0.04
Fat	0.04
Bone	0.04
Liver	0.13
Lung	0.04
Heart	0.11
Kidney	0.16
Spleen	0.18
Brain	0.12
Skin	0.11
Nerve	0.12
Pancreas	0.11
Eye	0.11
Muscle	0.52 (0.11)
Blood	0.60
Intestine	0.11

Table 3.5: Conductivity mean values for tissues at 100 Hz calculated from the investigation on resistivities of Faes et al. [76].

Tissue	Mean conductivity [S/m]
Bone	8e–9
Tibia cortical	5e–05
Tibia cancellous	0.02
Fat	0.03
Uterus	0.05
Breast	0.3
Liver	0.3
Skin	0.3
Spleen	0.3
Tongue	0.3
Kidney	0.5
Ovary	0.5
Thyroid	0.56
Lung	0.6
Muscle	0.6
Heart	0.6
Blood	0.7
Testis	0.7

Table 3.6: Conductivity of the whole and parts of the body obtained by integrating the conductivity values in Table 3.3 over various parts of the body, Gabriel et al. [67].

Frequency	Whole body	Head	Torso	Arm	Leg	Neck
50 Hz	0.216	0.254	0.223	0.195	0.196	
10 kHz	0.276	0.285	0.256		0.238	0.222
100 kHz	0.288	0.30	0.332		0.239	0.243

3.6.3 Estimation of effective conductivity

Different approaches have been found in literature followed in order to estimate theoretically the conductivity of tissues when no values are available. Peters et al. [62] took advantages of some properties of the tissues and proposed a strategy to estimate bounds for the conductivity values of tissues like cerebral cortex, liver and brain.

As described previously in Section 3.4.2, tissue can be thought as a whole of two components: extracellular fluid and intracellular space. In this sense, tissue can be considered as a suspension of cells, thus the effective conductivity of the tissue can be evaluated from the calculation of the effective conductivity of the cell suspension. Effective medium theories for dilute suspensions can be used to have an approximate analytical solution for the effective conductivity of a suspension of cells.

The cells are compounded by an external thin membrane and intracellular fluid (cytoplasm). Thus, the cell itself is heterogeneous. Despite this heterogeneity, the cell can be modelled by an effective conductivity that takes into account the conductivity and dimensions of both media. Considering a spherical cell with membrane thickness much smaller than the cell radius and taking into account that at low frequencies the conductivity of the cytoplasm and the membrane are equal to 0.5 S/m and 10^{-7} S/m, respectively, the equivalent conductivity of the cell results to be $\sigma_p = 2 \times 10^{-4}$ S/m [64].

Therefore, at ELF, the cells are treated as non-conductive particles and the intracellular fluid does not play any role in the conduction of currents. In this way, tissue is regarded as a suspension of non-conductive particles in an extracellular medium.

The extracellular medium is composed of water and ions. As the size of the ions is much smaller than the size of the cell, the medium can be modelled as a conducting continuum medium. Maxwell derived an equation (using the method of images) for the effective conductivity σ_f of a dilute suspension of spheres with conductivities σ_p in a medium of conductivity σ_m [77] as follows:

$$\frac{\sigma_m - \sigma_f}{2\sigma_m + \sigma_f} = p\frac{\sigma_m - \sigma_p}{2\sigma_m + \sigma_p}, \tag{3.8}$$

where p is the volume fraction of particles dispersed in the medium. This formula as described in reference [62] was extended for ellipsoidal particles, in this case all the particles have the same orientation and the applied field is along the a-axes of the particles, yielding the following equation:

$$\frac{\sigma_f - \sigma_p}{\sigma_m + \sigma_p}\left(\frac{\sigma_m}{\sigma_f}\right)^L = 1 - p, \tag{3.9}$$

where L is the depolarisation factor. After neglecting the conductivity of the cells yields the folowing:

$$\sigma_f \approx \sigma_m (1 - p)^s, \tag{3.10}$$

where $s = 1/(1 - L)^m$ is the cementation factor and depends on the shape and orientation of the particles, but not on the size. In this way, there are several sets of L_j^t for $j = 1$, 2 or 3, depending on the orientation and t indicating the shape of the particle, i.e. sphere, ellipsoids and disc. Due to lack of knowledge of details on the types of cells and micro-geometric structure, upper and lower bounds have been proposed. For elongated, homogeneously distributed, randomly oriented non-conducting spheres in suspension, Peters [62] derived the following expression:

$$\sigma_m (1 - p)^{5/3} < \sigma_{eff} < \sigma_m (1 - p)^{3/2}. \tag{3.11}$$

In this way, the resulting effective conductivity of the tissue is proportional to the conductivity of the extracellular fluid and increase with the volume fraction of extracellular fluid in the tissue.

In the human body as a whole, the total extracellular fluid is obtained by adding the interstitial fluid which surrounds cells plus blood plasma (blood is composed of plasma and red cells). From the International Commission of Radiological Protection (ICRP) publication [46], a relationship between extracellular fluid in the body $W_{extracellular}$ and total body water W_T for women and men has been extracted,

$$W_{extracellular} = 0.414W_T + 0.306. \tag{3.12}$$

The water content of the human body is generally associated to the fat-free mass or lean body mass, which refers to the mass of the body free of fat. Knowing that the water content of fat-free mass in adults is generally between 71% and 74%, for a person of 60 kg equation 3.12 gives a value of approximately 42% for the component of extracellular fluid.

Thus, roughly considering the human body as a whole, and making use of equation 3.11 for elongated, homogeneously distributed randomly orientated non-conducting spheroids in a conducting suspension with a value of 0.42 for the volume fraction of extracellular fluid and conductivity between 1.5 and 1.9 for the extracellular fluids, the conductivity of the whole body ranges between 0.41 and 0.52 S/m.

3.6.4 Dielectric data of the pregnant woman

In general for the female tissues, the data available can be obtained from the sources that have been described in the previous sections. For instance, if the study contemplates a detailed description, data can be extracted from the work of Gabriel in Table 3.3 which are generally used by many researchers or from Faes analysis of the data in Table 3.5. If the study uses pro-mediated values over some tissues, data can be extracted from Table 3.6. However, despite the abundant data available for woman tissues, except from the amniotic fluid, there are no available measurements for the human female organs during pregnancy at ELF. Therefore, as initial approximation the conductivity of the organs of the pregnant woman can be assumed to be equal to the conductivity of the organs of the non-pregnant one. However, for the placenta or umbilical cord, there are still no measurements available at ELF.

3.6.4.1 Amniotic fluid

The amniotic fluid, such as blood plasma or any other interstitial fluid, is a solution of electrolytes in water, thus its conductivity depends on the amount of ions in the solution and it increases with temperature. For blood plasma, interstitial fluid and cerebrospinal fluid measured values of conductivity at 37°C are available. Values of 1.58, 2 and 1.79 S/m, respectively, are found in literature. De Luca et al. [78] measured the dielectric properties of amniotic fluid at 20°C for different stages of pregnancy, observing that there is a significant change of conductivity related to the increment of the phospholipids concentration towards the end of normal pregnancies. Therefore, they obtained conductivity values that vary from 1.28 S/m until week 32 of gestation to 1.10 S/m at the end of gestation. Since the measurements have been performed at 20°C, a correction of 10% is carried out in order to evaluate the conductivity at 37°C, yielding values of 1.70 and 1.64 S/m, respectively.

3.6.4.2 Other maternal tissues

Based on the data reported by the ICRP reference values for anatomical and physiological data [46], the pregnant woman experiences many changes throughout gestation. Principally, there are strong changes in maternal body composition. On the one hand, the body mass increases, which is generated not only triggered by the increase of tissues enclosed in the uterus, i.e. the mass of the foetus, placenta and amniotic fluid basically, but also the body water and fat-content increase progressively. At the same time, changes in composition of tissues and fluids take place throughout pregnancy, such as changes in protein accumulation due to the enlargement of the uterus and mammary glands, changes in blood volume, as the blood plasma and red cells increase, and increase in the placenta, uterus and breast volume. Moreover, another physiological changes occur. For instance, basal metabolic rate increases throughout pregnancy, fluid intake increases during the first period of pregnancy. Respiratory function during pregnancy also changes due to various mechanical and biochemical factors, just to mention some changes. Finally, the blood-flow to the regions of the body changes markedly during pregnancy. Table 3.7 compares reference values for blood-flow to organs for a non-pregnant and a pregnant woman. It can be seen that, for instance, in the case of muscle, the blood-flow rate decreases from 12% to 8 % of cardiac output and there is no change in the mass of muscle during pregnancy, hence the decrease of blood present in the tissue may produce a variation on the muscle conductivity. On the other hand, for the uterus, according to Table 3.7, the blood-flow rate increases by 30 times and the mass increase is about 13.5 times as documented in the same ICPR article, since the mass of the uterus changes from 80 to 1100 g at the end of term. Consequently, an increase in conductivity may be expected, since the mass of extracellular fluid may increase.

Table 3.7: Reference values for blood flow rate to organs for the non-pregnant and pregnant woman near term, ICRP publication 89.

Tissue	Non-pregnant	Pregnant
Fat	8.5	7.8
Brain	12.0	8.8
Heart	5.0	3.7
Kidneys	17.0	16.6
Liver	27.0	20.0
Lungs	2.5	1.8
Muscle	12.0	8.8
Pancreas	1.0	0.7
Skeleton	5.0	3.7
Spleen	3.0	2.2
Gastro-intestinal tract	17.0	12.5
Thyroid	1.5	1.1
Uterus	0.4	12.0
Breast	0.4	3.5
Skin	5.0	8.7
Other	3.2	3.3
Cardiac output (1/min)	5.9	7.3

3.6.5 Dielectric data for the foetus

Due to ethic reasons, data for the conductivity of foetal tissues is still lacking and difficult to estimate since it is known that the conductivity of the foetal tissues changes during gestation as their constituents are changing and generating.

Lu et al. [79] measured the in vitro dielectric properties of foetal tissues in the frequency range from 100 kHz to 500 MHz. However, this data is not applicable for low frequency ranges. Kawai et al. [80] made measurements for rabbit foetuses at RF ranges. They also measured the conductivity of amniotic fluid for rabbits and compared with a human sample at 150 MHz, obtaining that the conductivity of the amniotic fluid is almost 1.8 times higher than the conductivity of muscle. For rabbit foetal tissues, they obtained conductivity values 1.3 times higher than the conductivity of muscle for an adult. Although this result is not applicable at ELF, it may establish a tendency of foetus tissues to be more conductive than adult tissues. This difference in conductivity values are in agreement with the results of Peyman et al. [81] which established that the conductivity decreases with age due to decreases in the water content in the tissues.

Figure 3.6 compares the water content of foetal tissues for different gestational stages and the proportion of extracellular fluids and intracellular space [82]. As can be seen in the figure, the water content of foetal tissues decreases progressively along gestation from 95% to 70% at term. However, concomitant with this regression, there is a redistribution of water from extracellular fluid to intracellular space. Hence, the volume fraction of extracellular space decreases along gestation from around 65% to 40% at term.

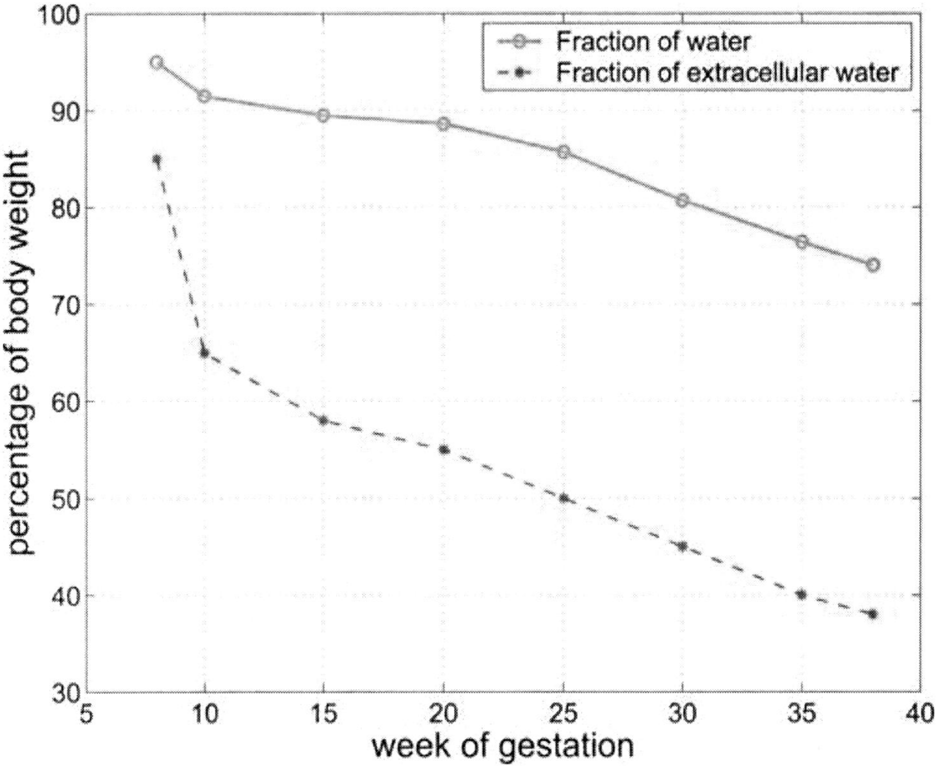

Figure 3.6: Water content and its distribution into extracellular and intracellular space along gestation [82].

Considering the foetus as a homogeneous conductor and its cells as elongated, homogeneously distributed, randomly oriented non-conducting spheres in suspension, Peters formulation can be used to estimate the effective conductivity of the foetus and making use of equation (3.9) upper and lower bounds for the conductivity have been calculated. Using conductivity values for the extracellular fluid σ_{ex} = 1.5 S/m, the lower bounds and upper bounds σ_{fL} and σ_{fU} are generated and using 1.9 S/m the respective lower and upper bounds are obtained. Dimbylow [49], based on the total water content of foetal tissues and making use of equation (3.8), calculated the ratio of conductivity between adult and foetus and then derived an estimation of the effective conductivity of foetal tissues from the adult's values.

Table 3.8 shows the results for the conductivity of foetal tissues calculated using the values proposed in this work and Peters method, together with the values proposed by Dimbylow, where p_s represents the proportion of solids in the foetus, σ_m the maternal conductivity and σ_f the foetal conductivity.

Table 3.8: Values of foetus conductivity proposed by Dimbylow and values proposed in this work. Conductivities in [S/m].

Method	Parameter	Week 8	Week 13	Week 26	Week 38
	p_s	0.05	0.90	0.14	0.260
Dimbylow	σ_m/σ_f	2.31	2.15	2.00	1.64
	σ_f	0.46	0.43	0.39	0.33
	p_{ex}	0.65	0.65	0.45	0.45
$\sigma_{ex} = 1.5$	σ_{fL}	0.73	0.73	0.39	0.45
	σ_{fH}	0.79	0.79	0.45	0.39
	p_{ex}	0.65	0.65	0.45	0.45
$\sigma_{ex} = 1.9$	σ_{fL}	0.93	0.93	0.50	0.50
	σ_{fH}	0.99	0.99	0.57	0.57

3.7 Summary

This chapter presented an introduction on the human body exposure to ELF electromagnetic fields. A general classification of the EM radiation according to its frequency, type of interaction with the biological tissues and consequent effects is introduced.

The differentiation between non-thermal and thermal effects is introduced. Dosimetry parameters and possible harmful effects at different frequencies are sketched.

The theoretical basis for the EM modelling of the problem of a human body exposed to an ELF field is presented. Departing from the macroscopic Maxwell equations for imperfect conductor material, the governing equations for ELF are derived. This formulation is restricted in frequency by the condition $\varphi\varepsilon/\sigma \ll 1$, i.e. up to a few kilohertz where electric fields and induced currents can be deduced from the solution of potential problems based on Laplace equation. Proper interface matching conditions between regions of different electrical properties including air-body are provided.

Finally, different sources of exposure to ELF fields and the typical levels of electric and magnetic fields that are frequently encountered under high-voltage distribution and transmission lines, near substations and in homes in UK are enumerated.

4

Numerical method

4.1 Introduction

This chapter provides a general overview of the BEM for potential equations, which is the basis of the numerical method of this work. In particular, the method is implemented for the solution of the ELF (Laplace equation) in 3D problems. A more detailed introduction to the BEM can be found in reference [82]. This work considers the direct BEM based on the collocation technique with domain decomposition. With the domain decomposition approach, non-homogeneous biological tissues can be represented as piece-wise homogeneous regions.

In general, there are two main technical bottlenecks in the computational aspects of collocation BEM [37, 83]. One of them is the pre-processing stage which involves the calculation of singular and near-singular integrals and their assembly into a consistent system of equations, and the other is the factorisation of such system of equations. This book introduces and develops a novel approach, named Staggered Boundary Element (S-BEM), for assembling the set of discrete boundary integral equations into the BEM linear system of equations, which improves the efficiency of the calculation. An efficient analytical method for computing the integration of the corresponding single and double layer potentials in the context of the S-BEM is also presented, with application to 3D potential problems.

Section 4.2 provides a summary of the integral formulation. Section 4.3 describes the boundary discretisation which yields a linear system of equations. Then, Section 4.4 shows the method employed for recovering the solution at internal points of the integration domain, as a post-processing stage, once the solution at the boundaries has been obtained. Section 4.5 describes continuous and discontinuous boundary element method. Section 4.6 summarises the main idea of the S-BEM approach. Section 4.7 derives an analytical method for the integrals involved in the S-BEM. Section 4.8 presents test examples in order to evaluate the accuracy and stability of the approach. The last test is oriented to problems of low-frequency electromagnetic compatibility, which is the targeting subject of the developed formulation. Finally, Section 4.9 provides the concluding remarks. The listing of some integral expressions is provided in Appendix A.

4.2 Integral formulation

The mathematical foundations for BEM have been known for nearly 100 years [37]. But it is only in the last few decades that the method has gained popularity for solving a wide number of problems described by partial differential equations (PDE).

The advantages of BEM are that it reduces the dimensionality of the PDE, thus requiring boundary-only discretisation, and that it is based on the fundamental solution of the leading partial differential operator, hence yielding high accuracy. In addition, mesh generation, pre-processing, infinite and semi-infinite domains are treated in a simple accurate way, and mesh discretisation is not necessary in planes of symmetry. The well-known disadvantages of BEM are that it is not good at solving non-linear and inhomogeneous problems, it requires the evaluation of singular integrals and due to the non-locality of the required operators, it yields dense non-symmetric linear systems of equations, which are often difficult to solve. Consider the following non-homogeneous Laplace-type equation:

$$\nabla \cdot [-\sigma \nabla u(\mathbf{x})] = 0, \quad \mathbf{x} \in \Omega \subseteq R^3, \tag{4.1}$$

where $\sigma \in \mathbb{R}$, Ω represents the integration sdomain, with any of Dirichlet, Neumann or Robin boundary conditions prescribed on the boundary $\Gamma = \partial\Omega$.

Partial integration by parts of equation (4.1), weighted by the free space Green's function of Laplace equation (u^*), leads to the following integral equation:

$$c(\mathbf{x}_s)u(\mathbf{x}_s) + \int_\Gamma q^* u \, d\Gamma - \int_\Gamma u^* q \, d\Gamma = 0. \tag{4.2}$$

The free space Green's function for a point source located at $\mathbf{x}_i$ satisfies the following equation:

$$\nabla^2 u^* + \delta(\mathbf{x} - \mathbf{x}_i) = 0. \tag{4.3}$$

For convenience the following notation is adopted: $q = \partial u / \partial \hat{n}$ [1], $q^* = \partial u^* / \partial \hat{n}$, where $\hat{n}$ is a unitary vector normal to the boundary Γ pointing in outward direction. In 3D problems, u^* and q^* become: $u^* = 1/(4\pi r)$ and $q^* = \mathbf{r} \cdot \hat{\mathbf{n}} / (4\pi r^3)$, respectively, where $\mathbf{r} = \mathbf{x} - \mathbf{x}_s$ and $r = |\mathbf{r}|$ is the distance between the field ($\mathbf{x}$) and source ($\mathbf{x}_s$) points.

The coefficient c in equation (4.2) is given by:

$$c(\mathbf{x}_i) = \begin{cases} 1, & \text{if } \mathbf{x}_i \in \Omega \\ 1/2, & \text{if } \mathbf{x}_i \in \Gamma \text{ (smooth boundary)} \end{cases}. \tag{4.4}$$

The integral expression (4.2) represents the starting point in the BEM solution procedure.

4.3 Boundary discretisation

The different terms in equation (4.2) involve only boundary integrals. The boundary Γ can be discretised into N_e boundary elements, so that

$$\Gamma = \bigcup_{j=1}^{N_e} \Gamma_j.$$

Each boundary element contains a number (N_f) of collocation nodes, where potentials (u) and fluxes (q) are evaluated. In the collocation approach, the values of u or q at any point, defined by the local coordinates $\boldsymbol{\xi} = \{(\xi_1, \xi_2) \in R^2\}$, on a given boundary element are expressed in terms of the corresponding values at the collocation nodes and the N_f interpolation functions ψ_k with $k = 1, \ldots, N_f$ in the following way:

$$u(\xi) = \sum_{k=1}^{N_f} \psi_k(\xi)\, u_k, \tag{4.5}$$

$$q(\xi) = \sum_{k=1}^{N_f} \psi_k(\xi)\, q_k. \tag{4.6}$$

By discretising the boundary and applying the collocation technique, expression (4.2) can be rewritten in the following way:

$$c(\mathbf{x}_i)u(\mathbf{x}_i) + \sum_{j=1}^{N_e} \sum_{k=1}^{N_{f(j)}} u_k \int_{\Gamma_j} q^*(r)\, \psi_k(\xi)\, d\Gamma_j(\xi),$$

$$-\sum_{j=1}^{N_e} \sum_{k=1}^{N_{f(j)}} q_k \int_{\Gamma_j} u^*(r)\, \psi_k(\xi)\, d\Gamma_j(\xi) = 0, \tag{4.7}$$

where the quantity $r = \|\mathbf{x}_i - \zeta\|$ is the distance between the source point and the integration point in the field element and

$$\varsigma = \sum_{k=1}^{N_f} \psi_k(\xi)\mathbf{x}_{gk}. \tag{4.8}$$

Here, $\mathbf{x}_{gk}$ for $k = 1, \ldots, N_f$ represents the coordinates of the geometrical nodes that define a boundary element, as shown in Figure 4.1.

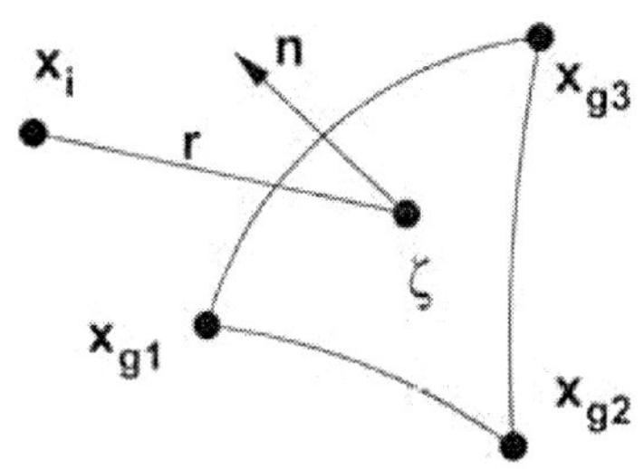

Figure 4.1: Distance between a source point $\mathbf{x}_i$ and an integration point ζ in a boundary element.

From a global point of view, N_b is the total number of collocation nodes in Γ. In the case of discontinuous elements $N_b = \Sigma_{j=1}^{N_e} N_f(j)$. When the source point $\mathbf{x}_s$ is located at the different collocation nodes along the boundary ($i = 1, \ldots, N_b$), the corresponding equation (4.7) written in terms of the global index l ($l = 1, \ldots, N_b$) can be assembled into the following matrix expression:

$$\mathbf{H}[\mathbf{u}] - \mathbf{G}[\mathbf{q}] = 0, \tag{4.9}$$

where

$$H_{il} = \delta_{il} c_i + \int_{\Gamma_j} \left. \frac{\partial u_i^*}{\partial n_j} \right|_{\xi_j} \psi_k(\xi_j) \mathrm{d}\Gamma_j, \tag{4.10}$$

$$G_{il} = \int_{\Gamma_j} u_i^*(\xi_j) \psi_k(\xi_j) \mathrm{d}\Gamma_j. \tag{4.11}$$

The global collocation node index $l = 1, \ldots, N_b$ is given as a function of the element index j and the local index denoting a collocation node in the element k, i.e. $l = \Xi(k, j)$, where Ξ represents a connectivity function. The boundary element $\mathrm{d}\Gamma_j$ is expressed in terms of the local coordinates (ξ) through the Jacobian of the transformation $|J|$ according to $\mathrm{d}\Gamma_j = |J|\, \mathrm{d}\xi_1 d\xi_2$.

Finally, the application of the prescribed boundary conditions leads to a determined system of equations of dimensions $N_b \times N_b$ of the form

$$\mathbf{AX} = b, \tag{4.12}$$

where the 1-column array of unknowns (**X**) contains the potentials and normal fluxes that were not prescribed as boundary conditions, the matrix A involves the coefficients of H and G and the right-hand side term involves the prescribed boundary conditions, multiplied by the corresponding **H** or **G** matrix elements.

4.3.1 Discontinuous elements

A physical mesh is mapped onto a logical one, which defines the computational space. The logical mesh is described by means of a table of 3D coordinates for each geometrical node in the mesh and a table of nodal connectivity for each element in the mesh. When the logical neighbourhood from the point of view of any element or node in the computational space remains constant it will be referred as *Structured Grids*, i.e. the number of nodes surrounding an element is always the same, as well as the number of elements surrounding a node, therefore the nodal connectivity can be expressed as a rectangular two-dimensional array, with N_e rows by N_{fn} columns.

Structured grids based on quadrilateral elements are desired whenever four-sided surfaces are present, since they help to minimise the total number of degrees of freedom. However, for surfaces other than four sided, as for example those containing holes or defined by many non-linear curves, an unstructured mesh with either triangular or quadrilateral elements becomes more convenient.

In case of discontinuous elements, this work considers both quadrilateral and triangular elements for the boundary discretisation, as shown in Figures 4.2 and 4.3. Details regarding local coordinates, interpolating and shape functions can be found in reference [84]. Discontinuous elements are easier to assemble in multi-domain BEM codes because each collocation node at the interface between two sub-domains will pose two unknowns (u and q), and two equations, i.e. one per adjacent sub-domain. Each element can be quadratic, constant or linear. However, as a rule of thumbs from experience, quadratic interpolating functions in purely discontinuous elements do not offer any advantage in problems with more than a few thousand degrees of freedom. Structured regions can be combined with unstructured ones, thus offering more flexibility when post-processing a complex geometry such as the one of the human body.

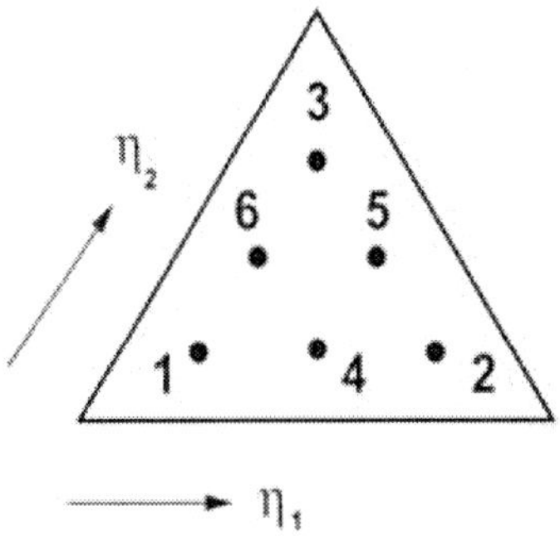

	η_1	η_2
1	1/4	1/4
2	3/4	1/4
3	1/4	3/4

Figure 4.2: Discontinuous triangular element used in this work.

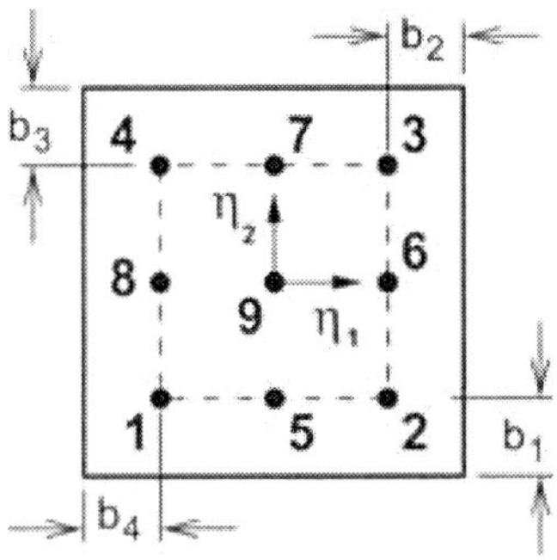

Figure 4.3: Discontinuous quadrilateral element used in this work.

4.4 Internal solution

Once equation (4.12) is solved, it is possible to obtain gradients ($\nabla u(\mathbf{x})$) and potentials $u(\mathbf{x})$ at any internal (observation) node $\mathbf{x}$ by means of the integral equation (4.2) and equation (4.4). In this way, the potential at $x \in \Omega$ becomes:

$$u(\mathbf{x}) = \sum_{j=1}^{N_e} \sum_{k=1}^{N_f^{(j)}} q_k \int_{\Gamma_j} u^*(\zeta, \mathbf{x})\ \psi_k\ \mathrm{d}\Gamma_j - u_k \int_{\Gamma_j} q^*(\zeta, \mathbf{x})\ \psi_k\ \mathrm{d}\Gamma_j, \tag{4.13}$$

and the gradient of the potential can be computed as follows:

$$\frac{\partial u\ (\mathbf{x})}{\partial x_p} = \sum_{j=1}^{N_e} \sum_{k=1}^{N_f^{(j)}} q_k \int_{\Gamma_j} \frac{\partial u^*}{\partial x_p}(\zeta, \mathbf{x})\ \psi_k\ \mathrm{d}\Gamma_j - u_k \int_{\Gamma_j} \frac{\partial q^*}{\partial x_p}(\zeta, \mathbf{x})\ \psi_k\ \mathrm{d}\Gamma_j. \tag{4.14}$$

where $\boldsymbol{\zeta} \in \Gamma_j$ specifies the integration point, and x_p is pth Cartesian component of the exploration point x, being index $p = 1$, 2 or 3. In the case of the kernel of Laplace equation in 3D:

$$\frac{\partial u^*}{\partial x_p} = \frac{r_p}{4\pi r^3}, \tag{4.15}$$

and

$$\frac{\partial q^*}{\partial x_p} = \frac{1}{4\pi}\left\{\frac{\hat{n}_p}{r^3} - \frac{3r_p(\mathbf{r}\cdot\boldsymbol{n})}{r^5}\right\}, \tag{4.16}$$

where $r_p = x_p - \zeta_p$, for $p = 1, 2, 3$.

4.5 Continuous and discontinuous boundary element method

Standard collocation BEM requires the discretisation of the boundary into a certain number of elements. Each element may hold either continuous or discontinuous freedom nodes, namely CFN or DFN, respectively. The former are useful for ensuring continuity of the potential at the edge between adjacent elements, but are inconvenient for expressing their normal derivatives, especially when the adjacent elements have different normals or in the case of unstructured meshes with multi-domain approach when many elements may share the same edge. On the other hand, discontinuous elements avoid these problems and simplify the assembly of BEM equations, but at the same time they spoil the continuity of the potential at the edges and usually create more than necessary degrees of freedom, thus becoming more prone to yield larger ill-conditioned systems of equations. Hence, the S-BEM proposed in this work is aimed to address this issue, by combining in the same element CFN for the potential and DFN for its normal derivatives.

In the field of singular integrals, different approaches have been proposed, such as regularisation techniques and the use of different analytical transformations to reduce the order of the singularity, numerical quadrature or refinement and partition of elements close to the singularity. References [85–87] compile recent achievements in the calculation of singular integrals for BEM. Particularly, Guiggiani et al. [88, 89] developed a general framework for describing integrals with any order of singularity, showing at the same time that no unbounded terms arise in the BEM when proper limiting process is performed near the singularity. Salvadori [90] proposed an efficient analytical approach for elasticity problems. Recent contributions of Gao [91, 92] provide the theory and a self-contained Fortran code for evaluating regular and singular integrals in BEM using numerical quadratures. In particular, the case of integrating the single and double layer potentials of Laplacian kernel over either flat linear or flat constant 3D elements allows analytical treatment, and does not require the use of numerical quadratures, which are efficient for regular integrations but normally tend to increase the computational burden and become inaccurate when the source point becomes too close to the boundary. An original approach in analytical integration schemes was proposed by Medina and Liggett [93]. It is worth mentioning that integration of $1/r$-type kernels in flat elements for 3D problems represents a subset in the already well-established literature. However to obtain the closed analytical results involves rather tedious algebraic manipulation and to the best of the author's knowledge, the final results are not extensively spread in the literature. Hence, this work includes the analytical development and wraps the corresponding methodology in a self-contained tested computer code. The motivation arises from the need to improve the accuracy of the calculation in complex geometries which involve large number of degrees of freedom and very dissimilar sizes of boundary elements and to minimise as much as possible the computational time in the pre-processing stage. The approach for singular integrals used in this work is a continuation of the works of Allgower and Kalik [94] on the computation of nearly singular integrals and Srivastava and Contractor [95]. The evaluation of the works of Hayami [96] for numerical quadratures in curved elements, Ma and Kamiya [97], Zhongrong et al. [98] has also been taken into account.

4.6 Staggered boundary element

The S-BEM is a collocation approach which employs a combined continuous–discontinuous element for boundary discretisation in which potentials u are associated to CFNs only, while normal derivatives q are associated to DFNs only. To illustrate the motivation of this approach, consider solving equation (4.1) in a multi-domain scheme where σ is piece-wise continuous across sub-regions inside the cube shown in Figure 4.4, thus requiring non-structured multi-domain mesh where each sub-domain is represented by a tetrahedron (tet) of different σ. Tet A is formed by continuous nodes 1, 2, 3, 4, whereas B is formed by nodes 2, 3, 4, 5. A and B share the triangular boundary element defined by nodes 2, 3 and 4 as common interface. Then, the advantage of a staggered assignment of potentials and normal derivatives can be appreciated when assembling the multi-domain 3D problem in which the equations of continuity of normal fluxes $q = -\sigma\nabla u \cdot \hat{\mathbf{n}}$ are prescribed across the internal interface, i.e. central node '0' in Figure 4.4 and continuity of potentials u is ensured at corner points 2, 3 and 4. The problem of using CFNs for normal fluxes in 3D problems with unstructured meshes[2] is that many different sub-domains and faces may share a common CFN thus complicating the assembly scheme of the BEM equations and causing unbalanced system of equations. Taigbenu [99] has successfully worked out an elegant solution for the 2D Green Element Method (GEM) [100] by assigning the potential and all the normal fluxes coming from the adjacent edges to the same CFN as seen in Figure 4.5. In this case, the central node introduces six unknowns (one potential and five normal fluxes), but at the same time it prescribes six equations, one BEM equation per each sub-domain plus an equation for conservation of flux given by: $\Sigma q_i \Delta\beta_i = 0$, where $\Delta\beta_i$ is the angle between faces of ith sub-domain. Therefore, the system becomes naturally balanced. However, in unstructured 3D GEM, the benefits of this approach are in principle lost, since not only the number of equations and unknowns differ from point to point thus probably yielding ill-conditioned systems, but also the number of degrees of freedom might become unnecessarily large. Ramsak et al. [101] have introduced a novel continuous–discontinuous node distribution for 2D problems in unsteady laminar flow calculations.

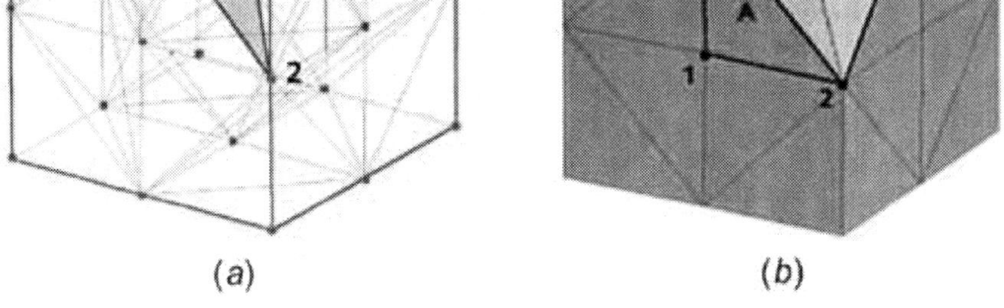

Figure 4.4: (a) Example of a multi-domain problem with 26 continuous nodes and 44 tetrahedral sub-domains. (b) Interface defined by nodes 2, 3, 4 is shared between sub-domains A and B.

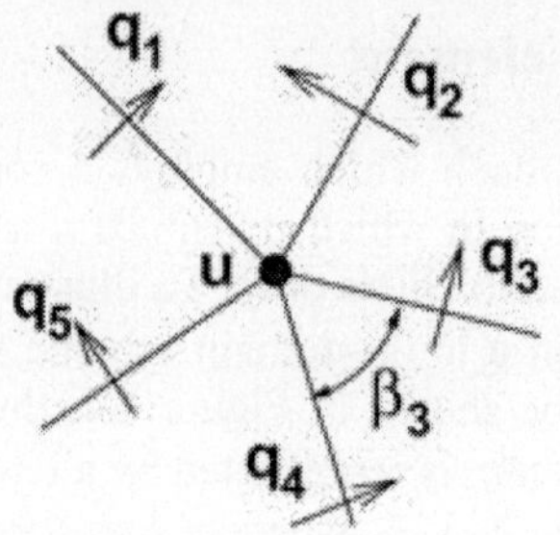

Figure 4.5: Assignment of degrees of freedom in the 2D GEM.

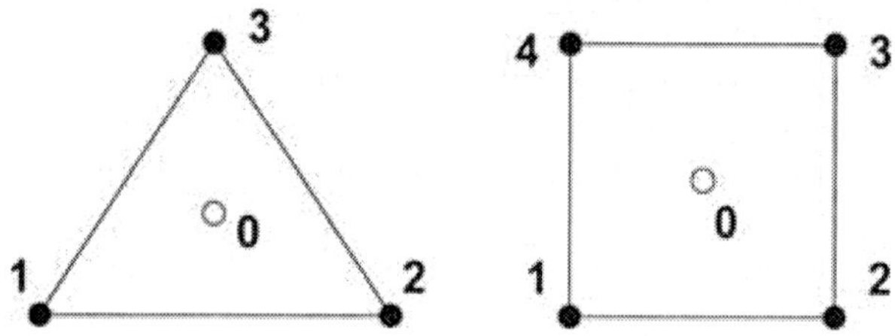

Figure 4.6: Staggered linear-constant triangular and quadrilateral boundary elements. The continuous nodes 1 to 4 are used to interpolate the potential u, whereas node 0 is used to interpolate the normal derivative q for the whole element.

In order to solve equation (4.2), Γ is discretised into N_e S-BEM Γ_e as shown in Figure 4.6. In this example, q is considered constant throughout Γ_e by means of one discontinuous collocation node in the centroid of the element (node 0) and u is linearly represented by means of CFNs at the vertices[3] such that:

$$u = \sum_{a=1}^{3} N_a(\eta_1, \eta_2) u_a, \tag{4.17}$$

where $a = 1, 2, 3$ denotes one of the CFNs, u_a is the potential at the collocation nodes, $N_a(\eta_1, \eta_2)$ are the corresponding interpolating functions and (η_1, η_2) denotes the local coordinates of the field point. In a general S-BEM, the interpolation degree for u or q can be different. In addition, the interpolation degree for the shape functions describing the geometry can be independent as well. In particular, this work deals with the linear-constant-linear combination, for potential, flux and geometry, respectively in a triangular element, but the idea of staggered element can be extended to any combination. Thus, the discretised boundary integral equation for triangular elements becomes:

$$c_s u_s + \sum_{e=1}^{N_e} \sum_{a=1}^{3} h^{(e,a)} u_{e,a} - \sum_{e=1}^{N_e} g^{(e)} q_e = 0, \tag{4.18}$$

where $u_{e,a}$ is the potential at the ath CFN in the eth element, q_e is the mean normal flux at central DFN of eth element, and $g^{(e)}$ and $h^{(e,a)}$ are the following S-BEM integrals to be computed in the next section:

$$g^{(e)} = \frac{1}{4\pi} \int_{\Gamma_e} \frac{1}{r} \mathrm{d}\Gamma_e, \tag{4.19}$$

$$h^{(e,a)} = \frac{1}{4\pi} \int_{\Gamma_e} \frac{\mathbf{r} \cdot \mathbf{n}}{r^3} N_a \mathrm{d}\Gamma_e. \tag{4.20}$$

The assembly scheme consists in appending one equation (4.2) per each selected source point $\mathbf{x}_s$ per sub-domain, to the global system of equations ($\mathbf{Ax} = b$), where $\mathbf{A} \in R^{n \times m}$ contains the coefficients $h^{(e,a)}$ and $g^{(e)}$, $\mathbf{x}$ is a 1-column array with the unknown u and q, b is the right-hand-side 1-column array formed by the boundary conditions. The pseudocode in Figure 4.7 illustrates the assembly scheme, where Ω_s is a sub-domain in the given integration domain Ω and k points to a row number in the final system of equations. Note that the source point $\mathbf{x}_s$ is chosen to be a CFN (DFN), only if its u (q) was not previously imposed as a boundary condition. Moreover, each node with unknown u (q) can generate as many equations (i.e. rows in the system) as sub-domains adjacent to it. In the case of DFN with unknown q, this number can be either '1' or '2' for external or internal boundaries, respectively, while in the case of CFN with unknown u this number depends on the nodal connectivity of the discretisation mesh. Hence, in multi-domain problems, the S-BEM may produce more equations than degrees of freedom and the solving technique should be able to deal with this feature, i.e. by incorporating a Least Squares approximation.

```
k = 0
for all sub-domain Ω_s ∈ Ω do
  for all CFN(DFN) in Γ_s = ∂(Ω_s) do
    if u(q) is unknown in CFN(DFN) then
      k = k + 1
      x_s = coordinates of CFN(DFN)
      append eq. (4.2) in k-th row of system A x = b
    end if
  end for
end for
```

Figure 4.7: Assembly scheme in the S-BEM approach.

4.7 Analytical approach for the integrals

This section presents the analytical approach for the integrals in equations (4.19) and (4.20). The analytical integration is considered for flat elements in order to improve the efficiency and accuracy of the pre-processing with respect to the standard Gauss quadrature approach. The method expresses the integrand in local polar coordinates, in order to reduce the order of the singularity. The integration is done first in the radial coordinate and then in the angular one. The former integration is straightforward, while the latter requires further transformation in order to obtain a closed expression of practical use for its computational implementation. The derivation is next presented for the flat triangular staggered element shown in Figure 4.6.

The projection of the source point $\mathbf{x}_s$ onto the plane that contains Γ_e is given by $\mathbf{x}_0 = \mathbf{x}_s - c\,\mathbf{x}_0 = \mathbf{x}_s - c\hat{\mathbf{n}}$, where $c = (\mathbf{x}_s - \mathbf{v}_1)\cdot c = (\mathbf{x}_s - \mathbf{v}_1) \cdot \hat{\mathbf{n}}$, and $\mathbf{v}_k$ ($k = \{1, 2, 3\}$) are the geometrical nodes that describe the triangle shown in Figure 4.8.

A system of coordinates (local to Γ_e) is defined, centred at $\mathbf{x}_0$ with axes η_1, η_2, η_3 given by the following equation:

$$\hat{\eta}_1 = \frac{\mathbf{v}_2 - \mathbf{v}_1}{\| \mathbf{v}_2 - \mathbf{v}_1 \|}; \quad \hat{\eta}_3 = \frac{\hat{\eta}_1 \times (\mathbf{v}_3 - \mathbf{v}_1)}{\| \mathbf{v}_3 - \mathbf{v}_1 \|}; \quad \hat{\eta}_2 = \hat{\eta}_3 \times \hat{\eta}_1. \tag{4.21}$$

Then, adopting cylindrical coordinates (ρ, θ) so that the integration point ($\mathbf{x}$) can be written as: $\mathbf{x} - \mathbf{x}_0 = \rho \cos\theta \hat{\eta}_1 + \rho \sin\theta \hat{\eta}_2$, the source point as: $\mathbf{x}_s = c\hat{\eta}_3$ and the Jacobian becomes $d\Gamma_e = \rho d\rho d\theta$.

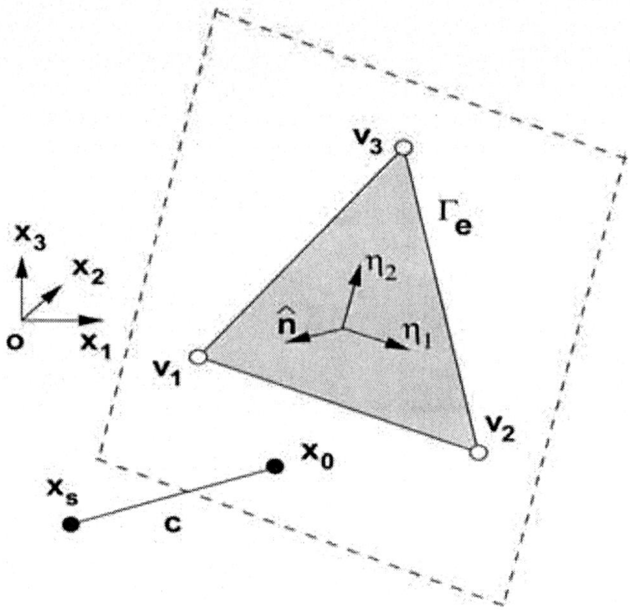

Figure 4.8: Source point $\mathbf{x}_s$ and field element Γ_e in 3D space.

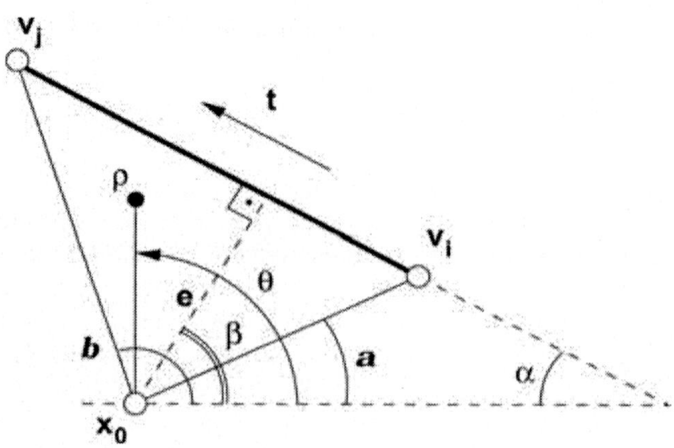

Figure 4.9: Parameters involved in the integration of region γ_i.

Integral (4.19) is then divided into N_s integrals, where N_s is the number of sides of the flat element (i.e. $N_s = 3$ for the triangle), according to the following equation:

$$g^{(e)} = \frac{1}{4\pi}\sum_{i=1}^{N_s} I\gamma_i, \tag{4.22}$$

where γi is the region enclosed by the triangle with vertices $\mathbf{x}_0$, $\mathbf{v}_i$, $\mathbf{v}_j$; $j = \text{up}(i, 3)$, the function up (i, N_s) is defined as the circular shift:

$$\text{up}(i,n) = \begin{cases} i+1; & \text{if } 1 \le i < N_s \\ 1; & \text{if } i < N_s \end{cases}, \tag{4.23}$$

and $I_{\gamma i}$ is defined as

$$I_{\gamma_i} = \int_{\gamma_i} \frac{1}{r} \mathrm{d}\gamma_i = \int_a^b \int_0^{R(\theta)} \frac{\rho\,\mathrm{d}\rho}{\sqrt{\rho^2 + c^2}} \mathrm{d}\theta, \tag{4.24}$$

being $R(\theta) = e/(\cos(\theta - \beta))$ and β is the angle formed between $\hat{\boldsymbol{\eta}}_1$ and the closest point of the ray connecting vertices $\mathbf{v}_i$ and $\mathbf{v}_j$ as shown in Figure 4.9. By considering equation (A1) from the appendix, it can be obtained:

$$I_{\gamma_i} = \int_{a-\beta}^{b-\beta} \sqrt{e^2[1+\tan^2\mu]+c^2}\ \mathrm{d}\mu - |c|(b-a), \tag{4.25}$$

where $\mu = \theta - \beta$ and e is the normal distance between $\mathbf{x}_0$ and the edge $\mathbf{v}_i\overline{\mathbf{v}}_j$. When $\mathbf{x}_0$ approaches to the edge, $\cos(\mu)$ tends to zero, and the integrand in equation (4.25) presents a peak-like behaviour which propagates large numerical errors in standard Gauss quadrature [86]. However, this problem is avoided by analytical means since as $\mathbf{x}_0$ approaches to the edge, the distance e decreases together with the area of γi. In order to integrate equation (4.25) analytically, the change of variables $t = e \tan \theta$ is proposed, where t can be considered as a coordinate along the edge $\mathbf{v}_i\overline{\mathbf{v}}_j$ so that $\mathrm{d}\mu = e/(e^2 + t^2)\mathrm{d}t$, and $R^2 = e^2 + t^2$. By using equation (A2), $I_{\gamma i}$ becomes:

$$I_{\gamma_i} = c \arctan\left(\frac{ct}{e\Lambda_1}\right) + e \log(t + \Lambda_1)\Big|_{t(a)}^{t(b)} - |c|(b-a); \quad (c \neq 0), \tag{4.26}$$

where $\Lambda_1 = \sqrt{c^2 + e^2 + t^2}$ and the integration limits are given by $t(a) = e \tan(a - \beta)$ and $t(b) = e \tan(b - \beta)$. The characteristic behaviour of the integrand $F(t) = c \arctan(ct/e\Lambda_1) + e \log(t + \Lambda_1)$ in equation (4.26) for different ratios between c, e and L, where $L = \|\mathbf{v}_i - \mathbf{v}_j\|$ is presented in Figure 4.10(a and b). The ratio c/L controls the derivative of F near $t = 0$, the smaller the ratio the steeper the derivative, while the ratio e/L has more influence in the asymptotic value of F. In the case $c = 0$ integral (4.26) becomes:

$$I_{\gamma_i} = \int_{a-\beta}^{b-\beta} \frac{e}{\cos\mu} \mathrm{d}\mu = 2e \operatorname{arctanh}\left[\tan\left(\frac{\mu}{2}\right)\right]_{a-\beta}^{b-\beta}. \tag{4.27}$$

The behaviour of the primitive of $I_{\gamma i}$ for $e = 1$ and $c = 0$ as function of the angular argument μ is shown in Figure 4.11. Note that when μ approaches to $\pm\pi/2$ a small error in the argument may introduce large errors in the primitive of $I_{\gamma i}$. However, in this case e becomes zero, thus cancelling the whole integral. Next, the calculation of $h^{(e,a)}$ matrix elements is shown. In the linear approximation, the interpolating functions (N_a) for the potential are given by $N_a(\eta_1, \eta_2) = v_a^0 + v_a^1\eta_1 + v_a^2\eta_2$, where coefficients v_a^k are the ones employed by standard Finite Element shape functions for linear triangular elements (see Appendix B). Therefore, the components of $h^{(e,a)}$ can be written as:

$$h^{(e,a)} = -\frac{c}{4\pi}[v_a^0 I^0 + v_a^1 I^1 + v_a^2 I^2], \tag{4.28}$$

where

$$I^0 = \int_{\Gamma_e} \frac{1}{r^3} \mathrm{d}\Gamma_e; \quad I^1 = \int_{\Gamma_e} \frac{\eta_1}{r^3} \mathrm{d}\Gamma_e; \quad I^2 = \int_{\Gamma_e} \frac{\eta_2}{r^3} \mathrm{d}\Gamma_e. \tag{4.29}$$

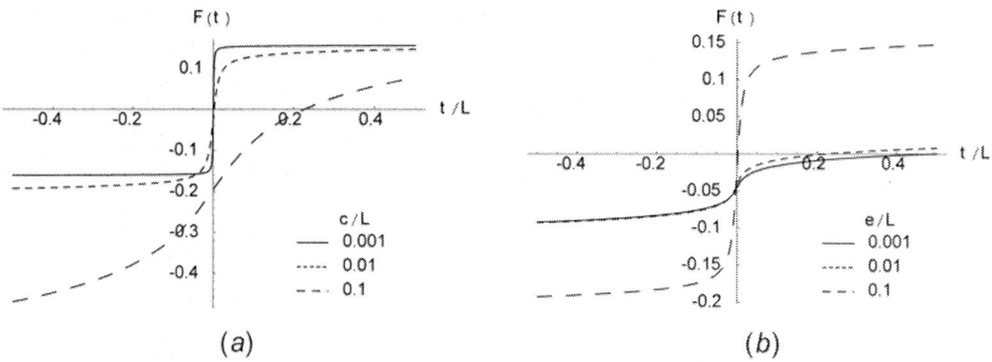

Figure 4.10: Behaviour of $F(t)$ for different locations of the source point relative to the field element of length L, by varying (a) c/L at constant $e/L = 0.01$ and (b) e/L at constant $c/L = 0.01$.

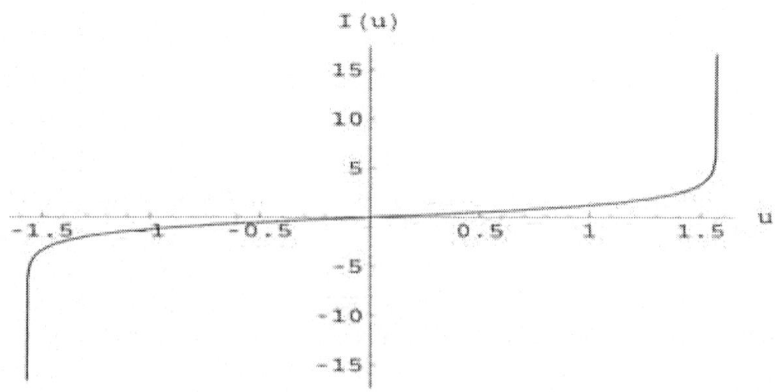

Figure 4.11: $I_{\gamma k}$ in function of angle u.

Same as before, decomposing the main integral into one integral I_γ^k per side in the following way: $I^k = \sum_{\gamma=1}^{N_s} I_\gamma^k$, where N_s is the number of sides in Γ_e and $k = 0, 1, 2$ denotes any of the integrals defined above. I_γ^1 can be written as follows:

$$I_\gamma^1 = \int_{\Gamma_e} \frac{\eta_1}{r^3} \mathrm{d}\Gamma_e = \int_a^b \cos\theta \int_0^{R(\theta)} \frac{\rho^2}{(\rho^2 + c^2)^{3/2}} \mathrm{d}\rho \mathrm{d}\theta. \tag{4.30}$$

By using equation (A3) from the Appendix for the radial integration, I_γ^1 becomes:

$$I_\gamma^1 = \int_a^b \left\{ \log\left[R(\theta) + \sqrt{c^2 + R(\theta)^2}\right] - \frac{R(\theta)}{\sqrt{c^2 + R(\theta)^2}} \right\} \cos\theta \mathrm{d}\theta - \log|c|(\sin b - \sin a). \tag{4.31}$$

The case of I_γ^2 is similar to I_γ^1 but replacing $\cos\theta$ by $\sin\theta$, same as in the previous section, by decomposing $\sin(\mu + \beta)$ and $\cos(\mu + \beta)$ and replacing the angular variable with $t(\theta) = e\tan\mu$ the following analytical solution is obtained:

$$I_\gamma^1 = \gamma_1 \cos\beta - \gamma_2 \sin\beta - \log|c|(\sin b - \sin a),$$

$$I_\gamma^2 = \gamma_1 \sin\beta - \gamma_2 \cos\beta - \log|c|(\cos b - \cos a),$$

where

$$\gamma_1 = e^2 \int_{t(a)}^{t(b)} \frac{\gamma(t)}{(e^2 + t^2)^{3/2}} \mathrm{d}t = [t\Lambda_3 - \Lambda_4]_{t(a)}^{t(b)}, \tag{4.32}$$

$$\gamma_2 = e \int_{t(a)}^{t(b)} \frac{t\,\gamma(t)}{(e^2 + t^2)^{3/2}} \mathrm{d}t = -e\Lambda_3 \Big|_{t(a)}^{t(b)}, \tag{4.33}$$

$$\gamma(t) = \log[\Lambda_2 + \Lambda_1] - \frac{\Lambda_2}{\Lambda_1}, \tag{4.34}$$

and

$$\Lambda_1 = \sqrt{c^2 + e^2 + t^2}; \quad \Lambda_2 = \sqrt{e^2 + t^2}; \quad \Lambda_3 = \frac{\log(\Lambda_1 + \Lambda_2)}{\Lambda_2}; \quad \Lambda_4 = \log(t + \Lambda_1). \tag{4.35}$$

The first term in the right-hand side of equation (4.28) involves the following:

$$I_\gamma^0 = \int_{\Gamma_e} \frac{1}{r^3} \mathrm{d}\Gamma_e = \int_a^b \int_0^{R(\theta)} \frac{\rho}{(\rho^2 + c^2)^{3/2}} \mathrm{d}\rho \mathrm{d}\theta. \tag{4.36}$$

Then, by using equation (A4), applying the usual change of variables $\theta \rightarrow t$ and using equation (A5) this last integral becomes

$$I_{\gamma}^{0} = \frac{b-a}{c} - \frac{1}{c}\left[\arctan\left(\frac{c\,t}{e\Lambda_1}\right)\right]_{t(a)}^{t(b)}. \tag{4.37}$$

Finally, it is worth mentioning that the described method can be extended to elements of any arbitrary number of sides, provided that they remain flat. Triangular elements are one of the most useful, as they are able to patch efficiently an arbitrary surface. Nevertheless, there are many situations in which quadrilateral elements become more efficient, i.e. they are especially useful for economising degrees of freedom in smoothly curved surfaces with nearly flat behaviour of the solution. For this reason, the described integration scheme has been adapted to constant-constant quad elements. However, quad elements for arbitrary surfaces tend to become non-coplanar (i.e. the geometrical nodes defining the element are not contained in the same plane) and in this case the presented integration scheme becomes inaccurate. In order to recover the precision of the method, the integral over the quad is sub-divided into triangular elements, as shown in Figure 4.12. The quad defined by nodes 1–4 is divided into triangles a, b, c and d which are integrated independently. This solution is easy to implement and allows a quick-fix to meshes containing non-flat quadrilateral elements, without needing to replace the analytical integration scheme by numerical quadratures.

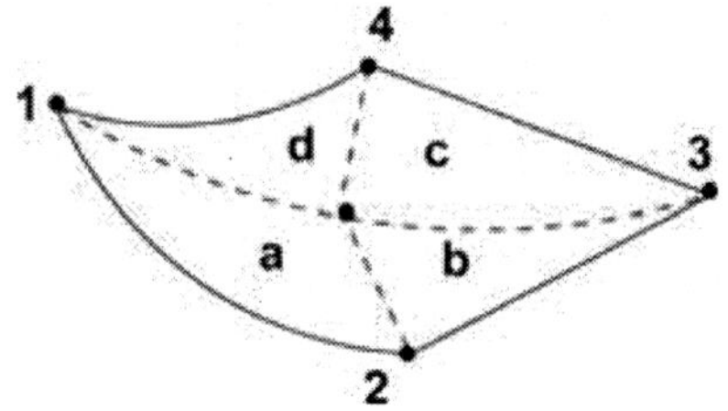

Figure 4.12: Sub-division scheme for non-coplanar quads.

In the next section, some numerical tests used to evaluate the accuracy and correct implementation of this scheme are resolved and discussed.

4.8 Accuracy tests

4.8.1 Example 1: Comparison of the S-BEM integrals against numerical quadrature

This example considers a flat continuous triangular element with linear interpolation functions, defined by three geometrical nodes of coordinates $\{x, y, z\}$ given by $\mathbf{x}_1 = \{0, 0, 0\}$, $\mathbf{x}_2 = \{1, 0, 0\}$, $\mathbf{x}_3 = \{0, 1, 0\}$. The source point, initially located at $\mathbf{x}_s = \{0.2, 0.2, 0.05\}$ moves to its final position $\mathbf{x}_s = \{0.2, 0.2, -0.05\}$ by varying c form +0.05 to –0.05 in 21 steps. The matrix elements $h^{(e,a)}$ and $g^{(e,0)}$ for this triangle have been computed with the developed analytical formulation and compared with an already validated BEM code based on standard Gaussian quadrature [84]. In the numerical scheme, the triangle is mapped onto a quadrilateral element, so that the integration is performed in a square domain employing 16 × 16 Gauss nodes. The comparison between analytical and numerical for the matrix element $h^{(e,1)}$ corresponding to node $\mathbf{x}_1$ is shown in Figure 4.13. It can be observed that the Gauss quadrature approach produces similar results to the analytical one as long as the source point is farther than at least five times the characteristic size of the field element. This lack of accuracy can be fixed by adding more Gauss points, however the computational cost increases. On the other hand, when the source point becomes closer to the field element, the analytical approach remains accurate without adding more complexity to the calculation.

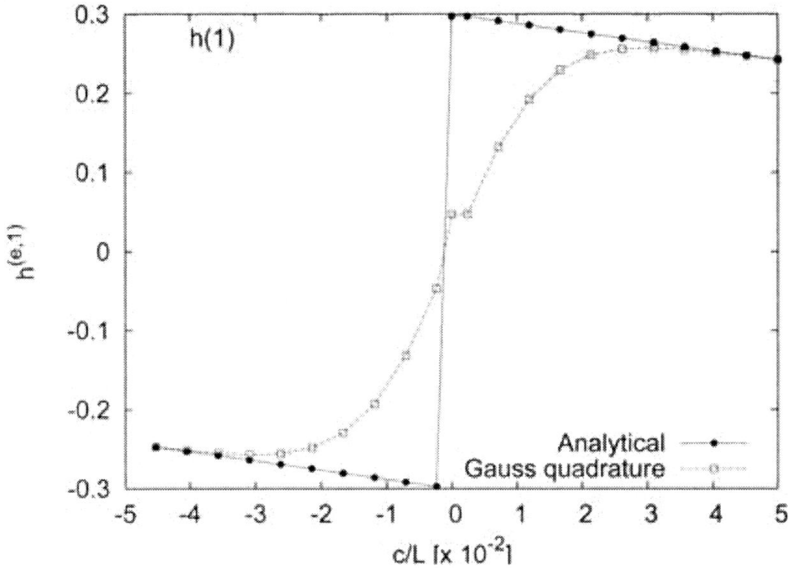

Figure 4.13: Comparison between Gauss quadrature (numerical) and developed analytical expression for $h^{(e,1)}$ component considered in Example 1, as the source point approaches the field element ($L = 1$ is the characteristic length of the element).

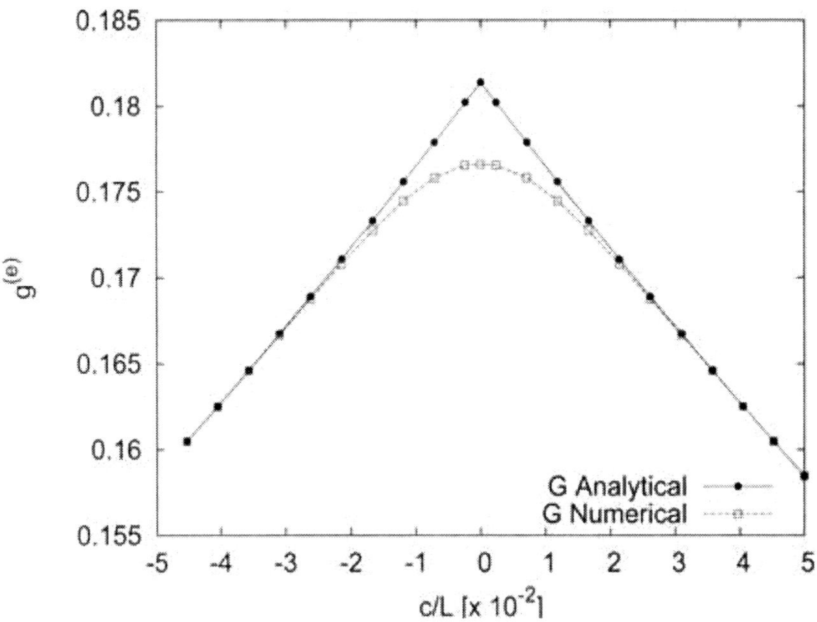

Figure 4.14: Comparison between Gauss quadrature (numerical) and the currently developed analytical expression for the integral of $1/r$ on a flat triangular element. ($L = 1$ is the characteristic length of the element).

Both results are in good agreement for c/L ratios larger than 3×10^{-2}. In addition, the figure illustrates the typical problem of inaccuracy in standard numerical integration schemes when c/L becomes too small (near-singular limit). This is the main advantage of analytical schemes for near-singular integrals, in addition to the reduction in the number of floating point iterations with respect to Gauss quadratures. Figure 4.14 shows a comparison between analytical and numerical results for the integral of $1/r$ over the above mentioned triangular element. Same as before, results are comparable until the near-singular limit when the numerical scheme looses accuracy.

A second comparison consists in shifting horizontally the source point at constant c from $\mathbf{x}_s = \{0.0, 0.1, c\}$ to $\mathbf{x}_s = \{1.0, 0.1, c\}$. This test has been repeated for different values of c and the results are shown in Figure 4.15 which compares the corresponding Gaussian quadrature with the analytical solution obtained in this work. The horizontal axis (Δx) ranging from 0 to 1 indicates the distance from the starting point. Results are comparable until Gauss quadrature becomes unstable at $c/L \lesssim 0.02$. This threshold can be improved either by increasing the number of Gauss points or by subdividing the element close to $\mathbf{x}_0$, but this will add more computational burden to the calculation.

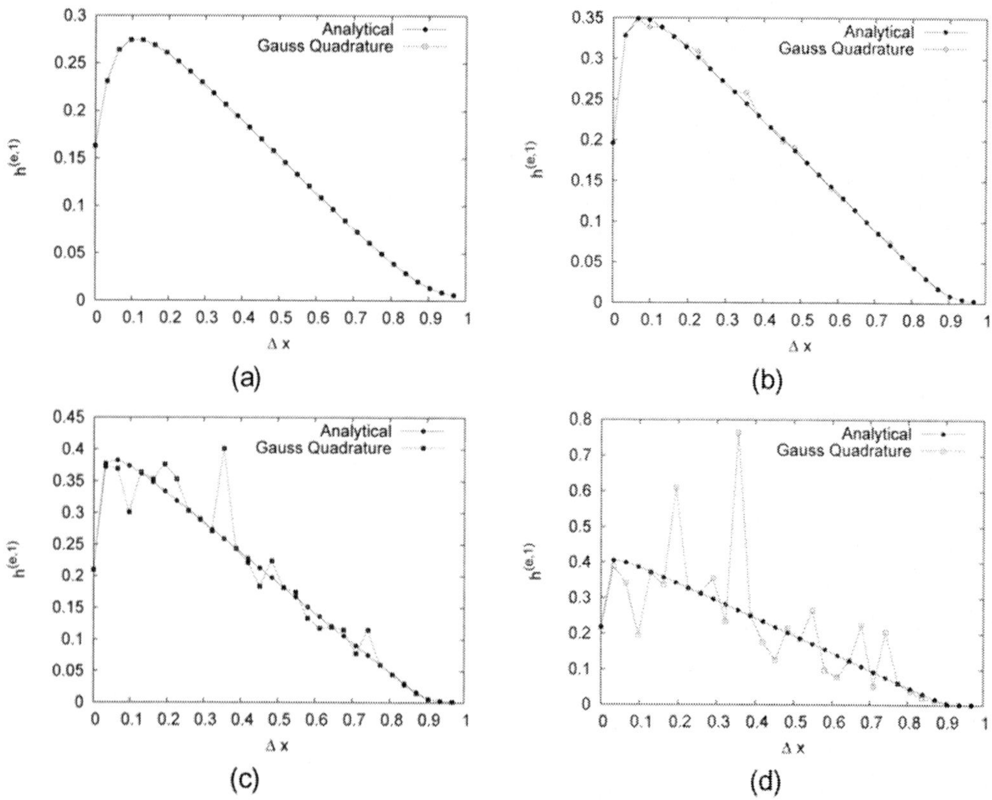

Figure 4.15: Evaluation of $h^{(e,1)}$ element when the source point moves horizontally over the triangle at different heights c. The numerical quadrature begins to fail when $\mathbf{x}_s$ approaches the element. (a) $c = 5E-2$; (b) $c = 2E-2$; (d) $c = 1E-2$; (e) $c = 5E-3$.

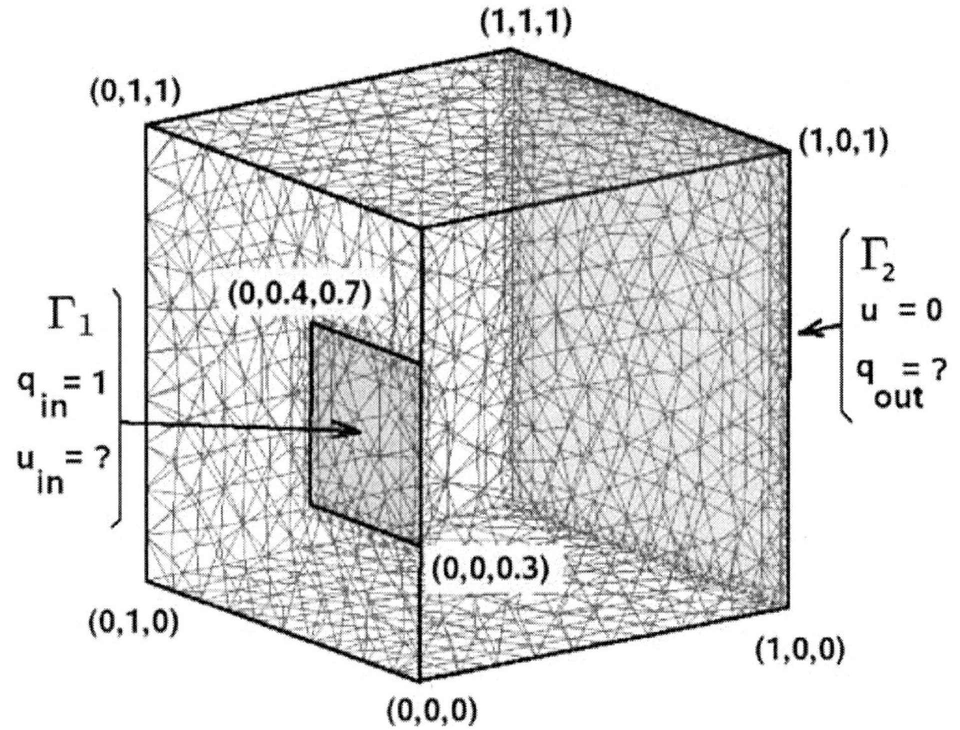

Figure 4.16: Dimensions and boundary conditions applied to the unitary cube in Example 2. The numbers between brackets indicate (x, y, z) coordinates.

4.8.2 Example 2: Mass conservation in a unitary cube

The accuracy of the S-BEM has been tested in many simple examples involving unitary cubes and Laplace equation. In order to test the accuracy of the S-BEM this example solves equation 4.1 in a unitary cube of dimensions $1 \times 1 \times 1$ with $k = 1$. Figure 4.16 shows the applied boundary conditions and the relevant dimensions of the geometry. A normal flux $q_{\text{in}} = 1$ is applied as boundary condition in a reduced surface Γ_1 of dimension 0.4 in width by 0.4 long at the front face of the cube with its lower right corner located at $\{x, y, z\} = \{0, 0.3, 0.0\}$. Dirichlet condition $u = 0$ is imposed in the back surface (Γ_2 at $z = 1$) and the unknown normal flux q_{out} is sought. All the rest of the surfaces were assigned adiabatic condition $q = 0$. The test consists in measuring to which extent the conservation of total flux is preserved by computing the following error between the inlet flux $Q_{\text{in}} = 0.4 \times 0.4 \times q_{\text{in}} = 0.16$ and the outlet flux $Q_{\text{out}} = \int_{\Gamma_2} q_{\text{out}} \, d\Gamma_2$:

$$\varepsilon = \left| \frac{Q_{out} - Q_{in}}{Q_{in}} \right| = 6.25 \left| \sum_{i \in \Gamma_2} q_{\text{out},i} A_i - 0.16 \right|. \tag{4.38}$$

where A_i is the area of each triangular element in Γ_2 and $q_{\text{out},i}$ is the normal flux computed by numerical approach. The problem was solved with three different collocation BEM techniques: (i) S-BEM presented in this work, (ii) 'BEM-0' with constant triangular elements in which one freedom node at the centroid of the triangle is used for representing both u and q and (iii) 'BEM-1' which employs linear discontinuous iso-parametric triangular elements with six freedom nodes per element. The last two methods were extensively tested in the past [84] and successfully used in recent works [102], therefore considered as reference in this present work. In this work, both BEM-0 and BEM-1 employ standard Gauss integration technique with up to 16×16 Gauss points for the integral in each element and element subdivision was employed in the case of near-singular integrals. The test was run for different refined meshes, and their computing times and errors were compared. The discretisation mesh and the linear solver (Lapack [103]) were the same for the three methods. Table 4.1 compares the performance of the three methods for four different meshes. The columns are as follows: N_e indicates the number of triangles in the mesh, N_{DOF} is the number of degrees of freedom produced by each method,[4] t_1 is the solver time obtained with Lapack [103], t_2 is the time employed to compute and assemble the BEM integrals, and ε is the error computed from equation (4.38). The normal flux obtained at the back surface is shown in Figure 4.17. The test was conducted in a PC Pentium 4 3 GHz, 512 MB RAM memory with g95 Fortran compiler running Linux (kernel 2.6) operating system. In all cases, the pre-processing time is smaller for the S-BEM due to the efficient analytical approach of the integrals. On the other hand, for the same degree of refinement (N_e), the number of degrees of freedom produced by S-BEM is smaller than the other two. This is roughly correlated with the shorter solving time t_1 achieved. In all cases, the error decreases with the mesh refinement and BEM-1 yields smaller error for the same triangulation. This was to be expected in view of the large number of degrees of freedom produced. However, when the comparison is done at similar numbers of degrees of freedom, the error, pre-processing and solving times are all significantly smaller in the S-BEM. Therefore, it becomes clear that S-BEM is more efficient than the other two traditional approaches, mainly because of its economisation in the number of degrees of freedom.

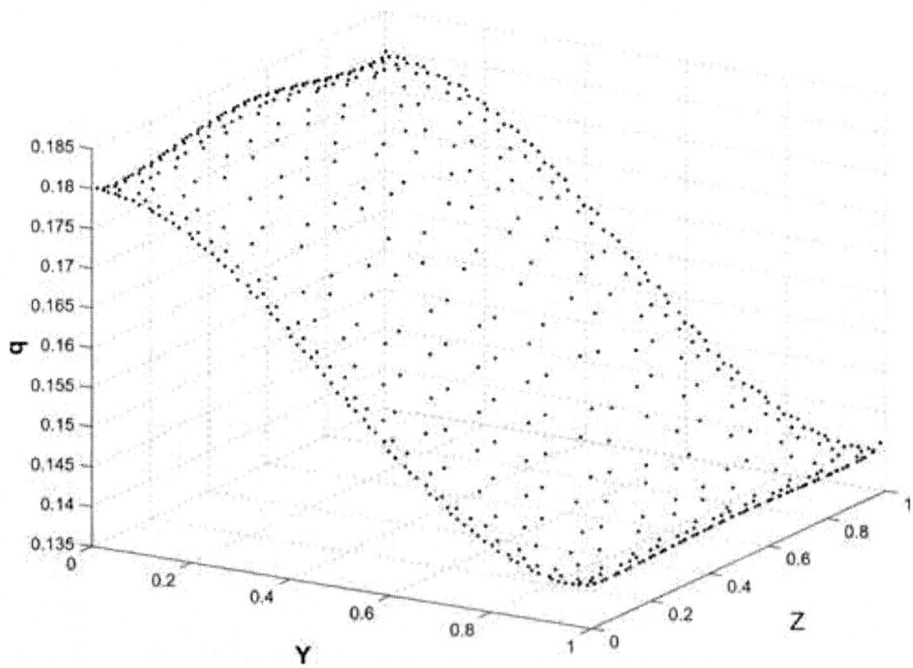

Figure 4.17: Normal flux distribution on the back face of the cube.

Table 4.1: Performance statistics for example 2. N_e = number of triangular elements used in the discretisation; N' = number of degrees of freedom; t_1 = solver time; t_2 = pre-processing time; ε = error defined in equation (4.38).

N_e	S-BEM				BEM constant				BEM linear disc.			
	N'	t_1 [s]	t_2 [s]	ε	N'	t_1 [s]	t_2 [s]	ε	N'	t_1 [s]	t_2 [s]	ε
320	177	0.04	1.1	4.1E-3	320	0.022	346	3.8E-3	960	0.81	115	1.1E-3
706	404	0.05	5.6	3.1E-4	706	0.29	171	1.2E-3	2118	15.6	582	6.4E-5
1238	704	0.35	20	2.8E-4	1238	2.23	553	1.4E-3	3714	85.6	2006	8.0E-5
2424	1408	4.10	70	7.9E-5	2424	23.4	2425	4.3E-4	7272	983	8598	1.8E-5

4.8.3 Validation for low-frequency electric fields induced in biological tissues

The developed application is oriented to problems of human exposure to ELF EM fields. In particular, current densities and EM fields induced in realistic models of the human body standing under power distribution lines. Hence, in order to test our approach with previously tested examples in this scope, ELF ellipsoidal model proposed by King [24] has been solved and the results have been compared with the analytical ones.

Time harmonic Maxwell's equations for imperfect conductors in ELF approach of characteristic length smaller than the propagation wavelength can be written as:

$$\nabla \cdot [(\sigma + i\omega\varepsilon)\mathbf{E}] = 0, \tag{4.39}$$

where $\omega = 2\pi f$, $i = \sqrt{-1}$, $\mathbf{E} = -\nabla\varphi$ is the electric field, σ the electrical conductivity of the body and ε the permittivity. The model representing a homogeneous biological tissue in air exposed to an ELF plane wave consists of an ellipsoid centred at the origin, defined by the following equation:

$$\frac{x^2}{a^2} + \frac{y^2}{b^2} + \frac{z^2}{c^2} = 1, \tag{4.40}$$

with $a = 0.3$ m, $b = 0.15$ m and $c = 0.875$ m, $\sigma = 0.5$ S/m and negligible permittivity, immersed in air with zero conductivity and $\varepsilon = \varepsilon_0 = 8.854 \times 10^{-12}$ F/m. The body is exposed to an incident electric field in $\hat{z}$ direction $\mathbf{E}^{inc} = E_0\hat{z}$ In the S-BEM model the ellipsoid is located inside a bounding box of dimension $L \times L \times L$, where $L = 8$ m. The boundary conditions applied to the bounding box are: U and $-U$ at the top and bottom surfaces, respectively, with $U = 4$ V so that to reproduce $E_0 = 1$ V/m. The lateral surfaces are all assigned zero normal component of electric field, i.e. $E \cdot \hat{n} = 0$. The model shown in Figure 4.18(a) with two sub-domains: one for the ellipsoid and the other for the surrounding dielectric media was discretised with an unstructured mesh of 1516 S-BEM triangles, yielding 2120 degrees of freedom. The electric field obtained inside the ellipsoid was $\mathbf{E}_b = (9.57 \pm 0.05) \times 10^{-8}$ V/m and the corresponding mean current density obtained was $\mathbf{j} = \sigma\mathbf{E} = 0.478A/m^2\hat{z}$. The results are comparable with the theoretical ones obtained in reference [24] as shown in Table 4.2. The mean value corresponds to an average between a random cloud distribution of observation points inside the ellipsoid of 100 points. Finally, the solution obtained with the S-BEM in the near field zone can be observed in Figure 4.18(b). The observation plane is oriented parallel to the z–y plane and contains the origin of coordinates.

Table 4.2: Comparison of electric field E_b and current density j_b results obtained with the S-BEM approach and the corresponding analytical solution [24].

	Analytical	S-BEM
E_b [V/m]	9.545×10^{-8}	9.57×10^{-8}
j_b [A/m^2]	0.477×10^{-7}	0.478×10^{-7}

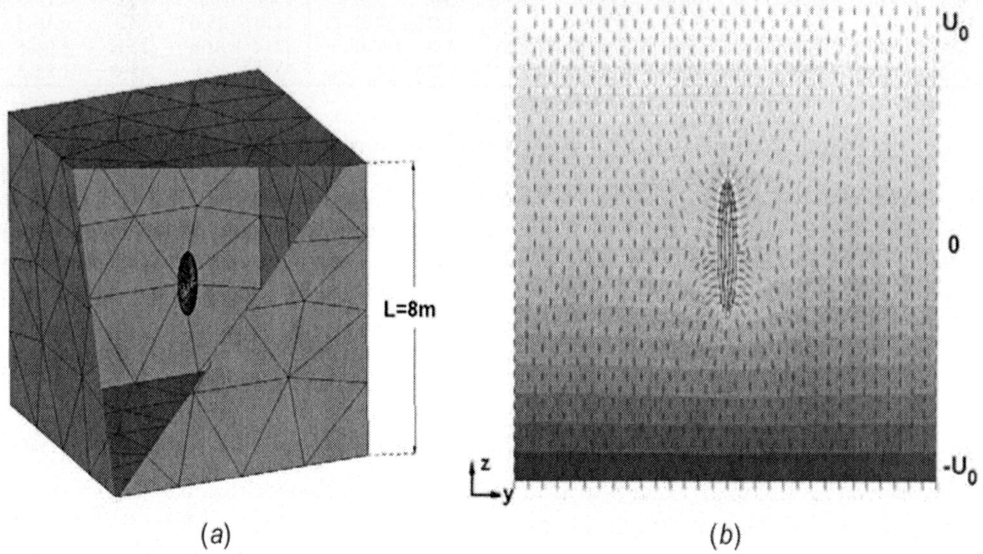

Figure 4.18: (a) Ellipsoidal model representing biological tissue exposed to an external ELF field. (b) Density plot of iso-potential surfaces and vector plot of the electric field in the near field, obtained with the S-BEM approach.

4.9 Summary

In this chapter, the general BEM has been outlined and a S-BEM approach for three-dimensional potential problems has been introduced together with the analytical derivation of the corresponding integrals involving the kernel of Laplace equation. The staggered assignment of potentials facilitates the assembly scheme especially in the case of multi-domain BEM with non-structured meshes. The main point of the staggered approach is to keep fluxes discontinuous and shared between elements, while retaining the continuity of the potential.

The presented approach is naturally free from the well-known problem of inaccuracy which appears when Gauss quadrature is directly applied and the source point approaches to the boundary element. When compared with other BEM collocation approaches employing unstructured triangular meshes, S-BEM results more efficient in terms of CPU time and error. Moreover, the assembly scheme retains the simplicity of a discontinuous technique.

The developed technique is efficient and reliable for solving electromagnetic compatibility problems in the low-frequency approach where Maxwell's equations can be decoupled into one Laplace and one Poisson equation.

Notes

1. q may also be referred to as a 'normal derivative', 'flux' or 'normal electric field'.
2. Unstructured meshes are preferred rather than structured ones since they can adapt more easily to complex geometry.
3. The continuous nodes are 1, 2 and 3 for the triangle or 1, 2, 3 and 4 for the quadrilateral.
4. Note that N_{DOF} for BEM-0 and BEM-1 are equal to N_e and $3 \times N_e$, respectively, while N_{DOF} in the S-BEM depends on both N
5. $_e$ and the particular nodal connectivity achieved by the unstructured surface mesh.

5

Exposure to overhead power lines

5.1 Introduction

This chapter studies the exposure to overhead power lines by means of the BEM. Although the dosimetry for this problem has been largely studied by detailed anatomy-based models using FDTD-like methods, due to the uncertainties in the definition of the tissue conductivity, it is still necessary to perform studies of sensibility to material properties variations.

Additionally, as the results have been shown to be strongly dependant on the external geometry of the body and organs, the aim of this study is to develop a parametric model of the human body, in order to easily vary external conditions and parameters of the geometry and study responses to that variations, as well as easily conduct studies of sensibility to material properties variations.

Therefore, the main objectives of this study are firstly to compare the numerical findings between conceptual models that take into account different degrees of geometrical detail, secondly to evaluate the influence of the relative position of the arms on the axial distribution of current density along the head and torso as well as along the arms and legs, then to compare the numerical findings between models which take into account the presence of some relevant organs and finally to analyse the influence of variations in the specification of tissue conductivity on the electric field induced in the body.

The chapter is divided into seven sections. Section 5.2 describes the physical model under study and the correspondent assumptions. Different conceptual models of the human body have been developed and applied in the numerical experiments performed. These are described in Section 5.3. Section 5.4 describes the aspects of the numerical implementation and different strategies applied in the numerical problem. Global results for the electric potential are shown in Section 5.5. Section 5.6 analyses the response of the current density to variations on the geometry of the conceptual model. Section 5.7 analyses the variation on the material properties and conductivities values ascribed to the different organs.

In all the cases, the induced current density computed in different conceptual models of the human body is analysed. As an ICNIRP/WHO workshop in 2004 [104], who investigated the potential health effects of physiological weak electric fields induced in the body at low frequencies, suggested that induced electric field rather than current density might be an appropriate dose quantity for effects bases on voltage-gated ion channels; results for induced electric field are also presented.

5.2 Physical model

This example considers a grounded human body standing below a high-voltage, three-phase, three-wire power transmission line with operating frequency of 60 Hz. The wires are located high enough to produce a uniform distribution of vertical electric field before getting close to the near field of the human body. Analytical expressions of electric fields generated by transmission lines without the presence of any conducting body can be found in reference [105].

In particular, for power lines above 20 m the vertical component E_z, which dominantly affects the induced currents in the body, can be considered as nearly uniform in the region $0 < z < 10$ m, $-5 < x(y) < 5$, when the wires are extended along $y(x)$ direction. Furthermore, a uniform electric field coming from the top onto a human being, will 'sense' its influence not before 4 m above the head. Figure 5.1(a) illustrates this situation. The equipotential lines in the air surrounding the body are nearly unaffected in the shaded area. The electric field along two vertical observation lines, one aligned with the standing man ($x = 0$ m) and the other 5 m away from him, has been calculated with a 2D BEM code in order to approach to the 3D model. The solution is plotted in Figure 5.1(b). By taking into account these assumptions and trying to minimise as much as possible the size of the integration domain thus reducing the computational cost in the 3D model, it is reasonable to adopt a parallelepiped, with height approximately 5 m and width 4 m as the unshaded region surrounding the human body shown in Figure 5.1(a). Hence, the 3D model considered has the dimensions shown in Figure 5.2.

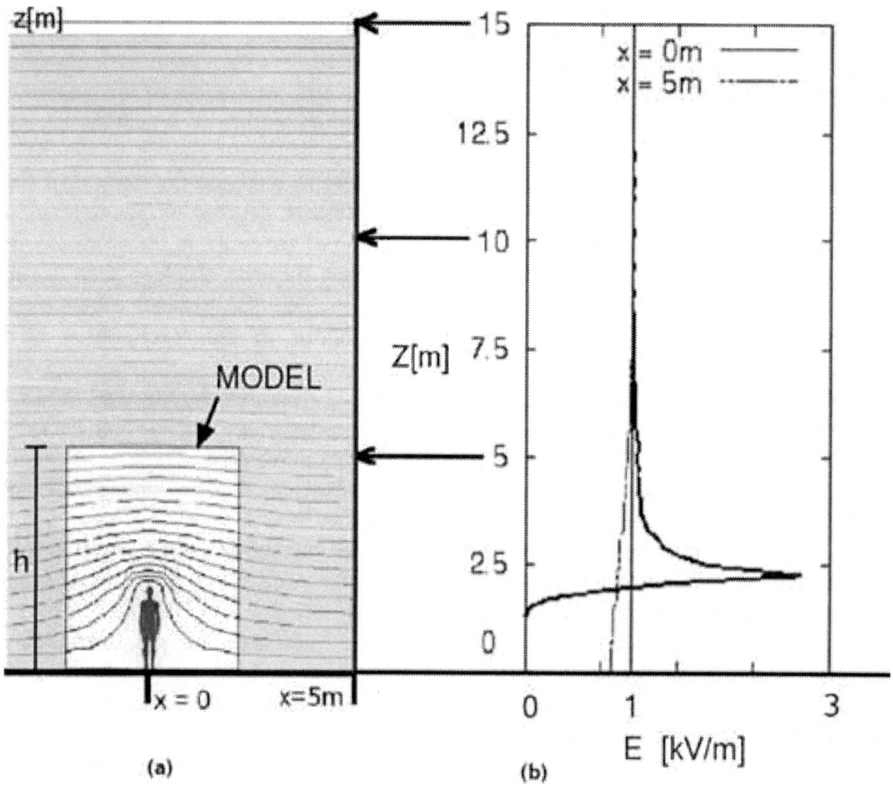

Figure 5.1: Electric field in air.

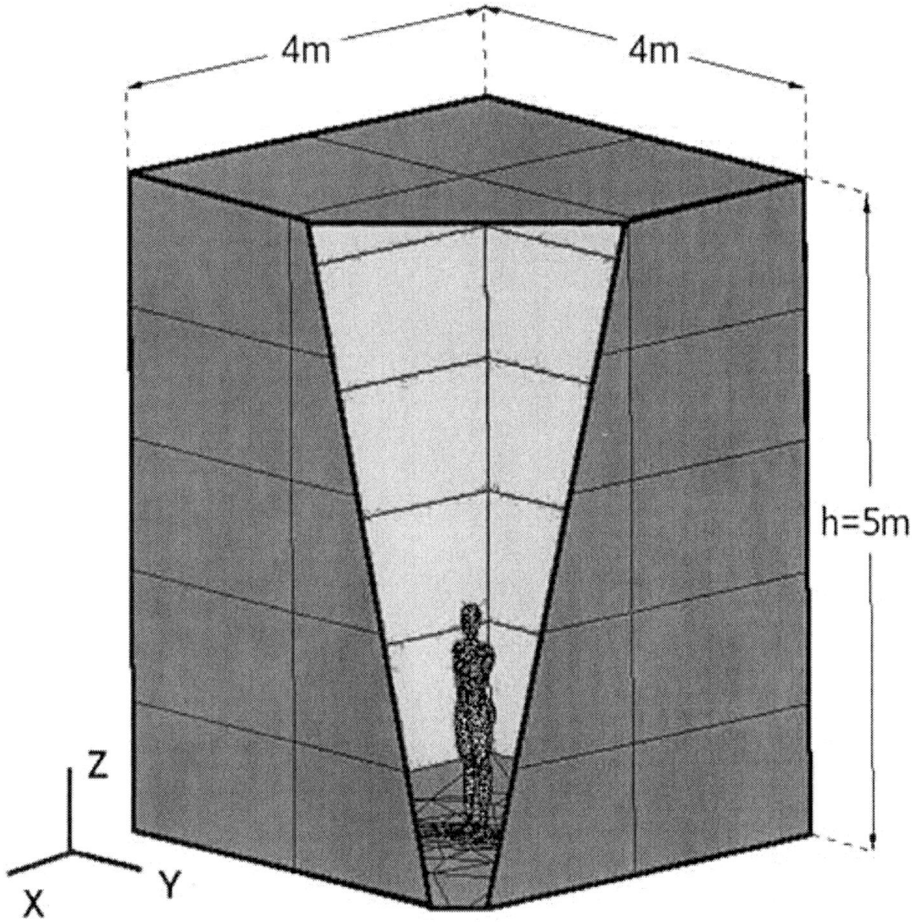

Figure 5.2: View of the integration domain in the near field. Distances are in meters.

5.3 Human body modelling

Basically, the human body was regarded as a saline fluid with conductivity $\sigma = 0.5$ S/m. Six different conceptual models of the realistic human body, namely CYL, HNA, HAO, HAU, HAD and HIO, have been developed in this work. Figure 5.3(a–e) summarises the main features of the conceptual models. CYL is a simplified model where the human body is represented by a cylinder of a diameter 0.364 m and height 1.75 m. HNA is a more realistic model, which considers the arms attached to the body as seen in Figure 5.3(c). The HAO, HAU and HAD models include the presence of arms and can be seen in Figures 5.3(a), (b) and (c), respectively. HAU considers arms extended making an angle of 60° with the horizontal plane. In the HAO model, the arms are extended parallel to the horizontal plane. HAD considers the arms down. HIO takes into account the presence of some relevant tissues like brain, eyes, heart, liver, kidneys and intestine. As a reference, in all the models the origin of the coordinates system is represented by the point 'O' of Figure 5.3(a).

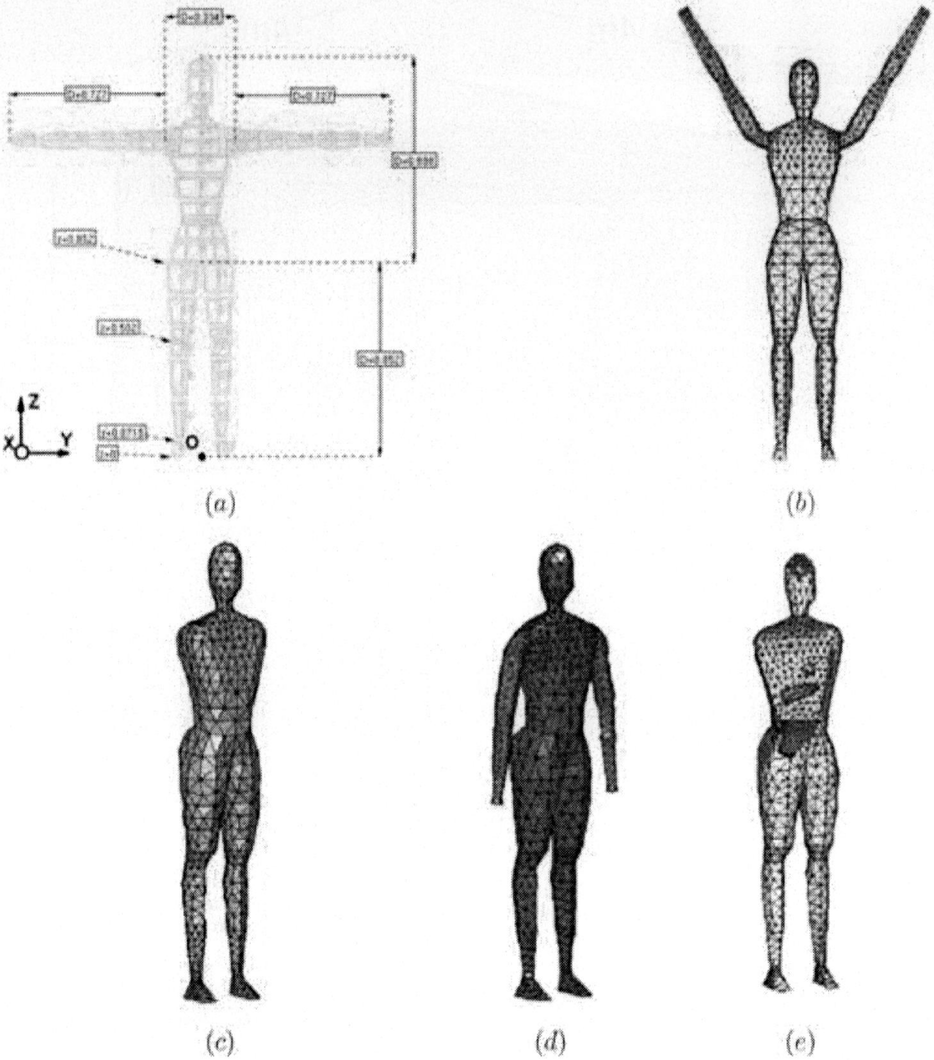

Figure 5.3: General features of the conceptual models for human body: (a) HAO, (b) HAU, (c) HNA, (d) HAD and (e) HIO.

The conductivity is considered homogeneous in all the models, except HIO. In order to model the different organs, sub-domains (or compartments) have been defined within the domain representing the human body. Therefore, all organs are treated as conductors embedded in a saline fluid with conductivity 0.5 S/m. Average values of physical and geometrical properties have been obtained from available databases and references.

A standard set of tissue conductivities has been used in this work and is summarised in Table 5.1. This set of values is used in the work of Gandhi et al. [25] and King [24, 106]. It is worth mentioning that the conductivities of the organs considered in this model by this set are relatively lower than its surrounding media.

Table 5.1: Tissue conductivities at ELF exposures.

Tissue type	Conductivity [S/m]
Muscle	0.5
Heart	0.11
Brain	0.12
Eye	0.11
Liver	0.13
Kidney	0.16
Intestine	0.16

For the sake of comparison and analysis, the set of conductivities proposed by Gabriel et al. [67] has also been used and examples will be considered in the following sections.

5.4 Numerical implementation. Extreme and minimal domain decomposition

In order to perform the discretisation of the domain and its consequent decomposition into sub-domains, two different numerical approaches have been considered in this work: Extreme and minimal domain decomposition, EDD and MDD, respectively.

In the EDD approach, the integration domain is discretised into an exuberant number of sub-domains. The motivation of this approach is to obtain a highly sparse linear system of equations in order to have the opportunity to use iterative matrix solvers. The advantage of iterative solvers over direct ones is that their calculation complexity is of the order of N^2 and their storage complexity is of the order of N, where N is the number of degrees of freedom in the system. In contrast, direct solvers require $O(N^3)$ floating point operations and $O(N^2)$ memory units for storage.

In the corresponding model, the domain has been divided into a hierarchical structure of layers of air and biological tissues yielding approximately 200 different domains. The number of elements generated ranges from 7000 to 18,000, depending on the geometry of the model that is considered. Because of the sparse pattern of the final system of equations, a family of iterative solvers were associated to this approach. In particular, the iterative conjugate gradient normal residues method from SPARSKIT2 [107, 108] showed the best efficiency.

A consequence of the high degree of domain decomposition in the EDD approach is the significant increase of intermediate interfaces, which introduce more degrees of freedom to the model, thus considerably increasing the size of the final system of equations.

In opposition to the EDD, the MDD approach attempts to minimise as much as possible the degree of decomposition, thus yielding more dense smaller matrices.

The motivation of this approach arises from the necessity to reduce the computational time and also to simplify the hierarchical order of the entities that define the geometry. This was carried out in order to simplify further modifications in the geometry of the human body, as for example the relative orientation of limbs, bending of the torso, etc. Domain decomposition in the MDD approach is performed only in the regions with different values of physical properties. The number of elements generated ranges approximately from 2000 to 3000. The linear systems of equations produced by the MDD have been solved by means of the linear Lapack solver [103].

Table 5.2 compares the discretisation statistics of the two different approaches described. The model that considers internal organs (HIO) and that without arms (HNA) are both shown as an example. As a concluding remark, conjugate gradient works better when the number of sub-domains is high, but when the number of volumes is low Lapack linear solver becomes more efficient and is able to reduce the computational time by a factor 3 to 4. For the case of the MDD approach, details on the meshes and computational times in a Pentium III PC with dual processors at 1GHz each are shown in Table 5.3, for which constant elements have been used, i.e. involving one collocation node at the centroid of the element. Figure 5.4 shows the CPU time versus the number of degrees of freedom of the system (N). A linear fit of the measured $\mathrm{CPU}_{\mathrm{time}}$ versus N has been performed with an exponential law of the form:

$$\mathrm{CPU}_{\mathrm{time}} = N^{a}, \tag{5.1}$$

where a is the parameter to be adjusted. The result obtained was an exponent $a \approx 2.2$, thus reflecting the typical behaviour of conjugate gradient based solvers.

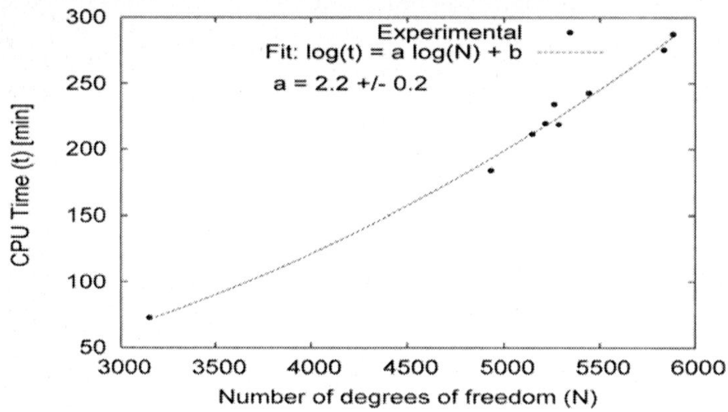

Figure 5.4: CPU time in function of number of degrees freedom.

Table 5.2: Statistics on numerical experiments for the different BEM models using constant elements

	HIO EDD	HIO MDD	HNA EDD	HNA MDD
Vol	179	8	52	2
Elems	16930	3496	6913	2646
NDof	32434	6646	12958	4946
	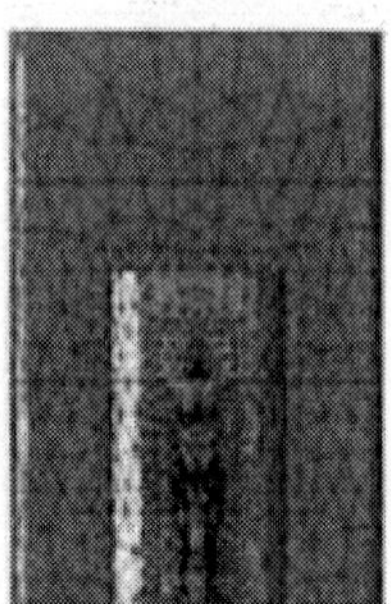	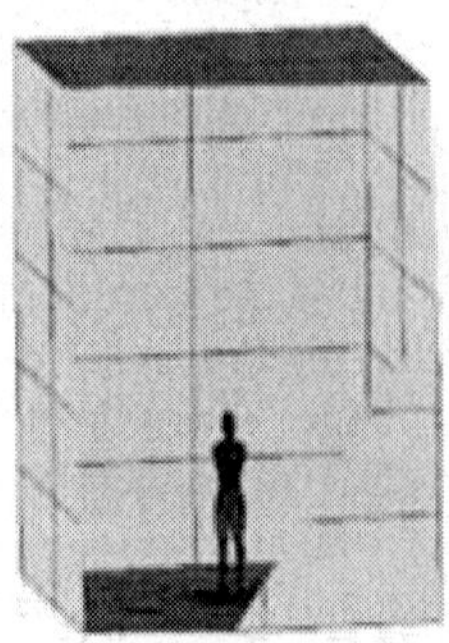	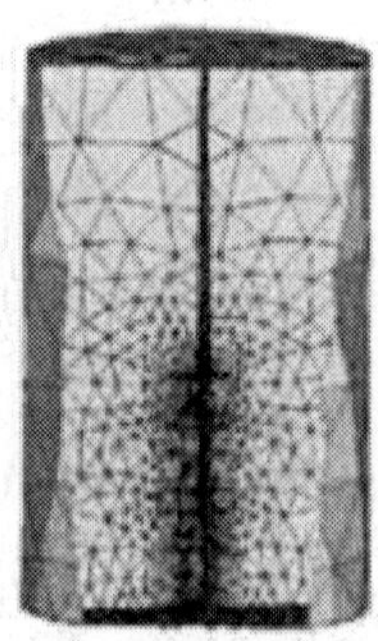	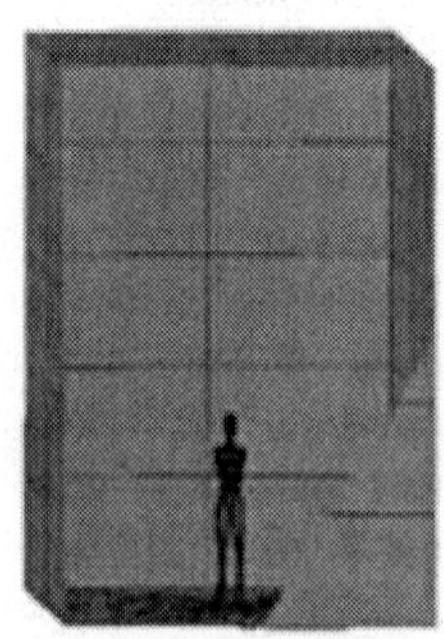

Table 5.3: Different models of human body solved with MDD and Lapack solver.

Model	Elems	Elems arm	Elems leg	NDof	CPU time [s]
	1845	96	184	3150	4378
	2736	493	434	5146	12,682
HAO	2807	624	359	5284	13,145
	3106	836	436	5886	17,243
HAD	2796	348	439	5260	14,069
	2631	406	365	4932	11,039
	2860	285	484	5214	13,200
HAU	2974	399	483	5442	14,577
	3082	850	434	5838	16,530

The results obtained with meshes having different number of elements have been compared for the cases of human models with arms. The computational time can be reduced by using both structured elements in appropriate regions of the domain and making the mesh coarser whenever possible.

5.5 Global results

Figure 5.5 shows the equipotential lines in the near field zone of the grounded human body for the model with no arms (HNA), exposed to reference incident field $E_z = 0.25$ V/m.

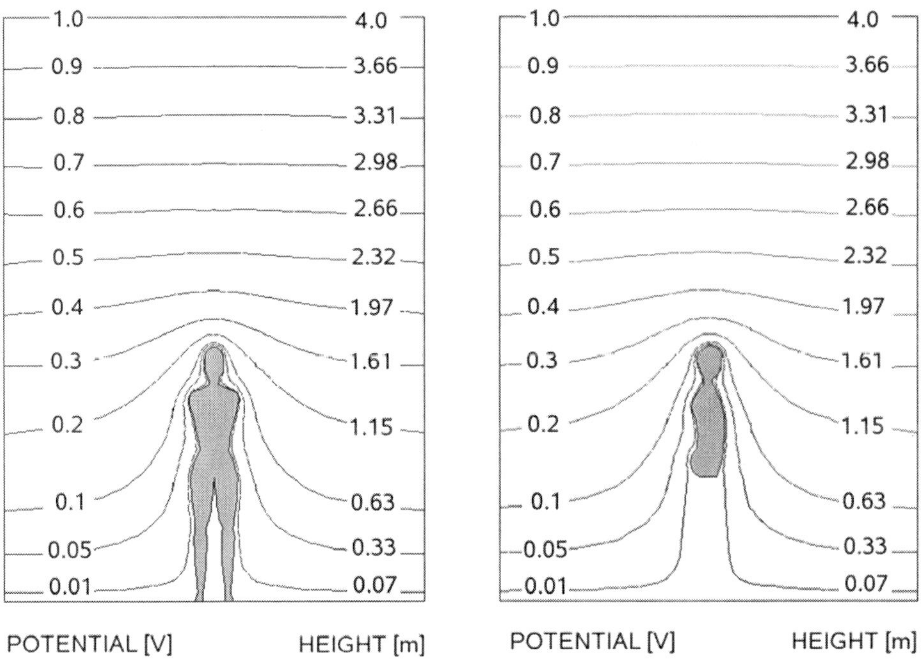

Figure 5.5: Front and lateral view of equipotential surfaces for the HNA model exposed to a reference incident field $E_z^i = 0.25$ V/m. The numbers on the left of each view indicate voltage, while the numbers on the right indicate height of the equipotential taken at 2.5 m away from the subject, i.e. when equipotential surfaces become parallel to the ground.

A 3D view of the HNA model showing the density plot of the scalar potential φ can be seen in Figure 5.6. For the numerical simulation, an absolute value $\varphi = 1.25$ V has been prescribed on the top surface of the model (i.e. at $z = 5$ m), whereas the bottom surface (grounded) has $\varphi = 0$ and the lateral surfaces of the model have zero normal component of electric field.

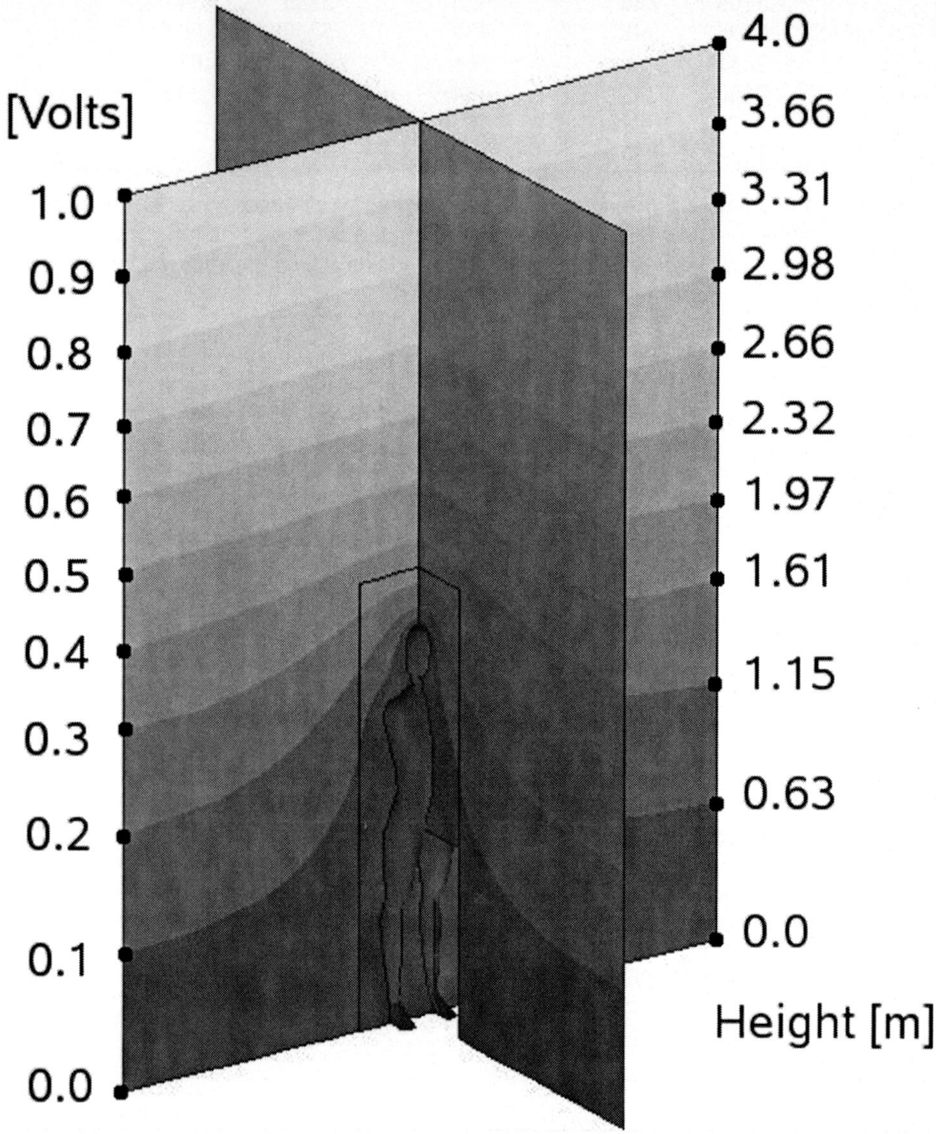

Figure 5.6: 3D view of the scaled results obtained in the near field for the HNA model. Unit potential has been applied to the top surface as boundary condition, i.e. the result corresponds to an incident electric field of $E_z^i = 0.25$ V/m.

A 3D view of the complete model with arms raised (HAU) showing the density plot of the scalar potential φ is shown in Figure 5.7. Owing to the linearity of the problem, the results can be re-scaled in order to obtain absolute potentials for any particular power distribution line higher than 20 m characterised by voltage and height. For example, in the case of a overhead power line that produces a uniform potential φh = 120 kV at h = 10 m height, the incident field at 5 m height is approximately 12 kV/m and the potentials shown in Figures 5.5–5.7 should be multiplied by the following scale factor k in order to obtain absolute values:

$$k = \frac{\varphi_h}{hE_z^i} = 4.8 \times 10^4 \tag{5.2}$$

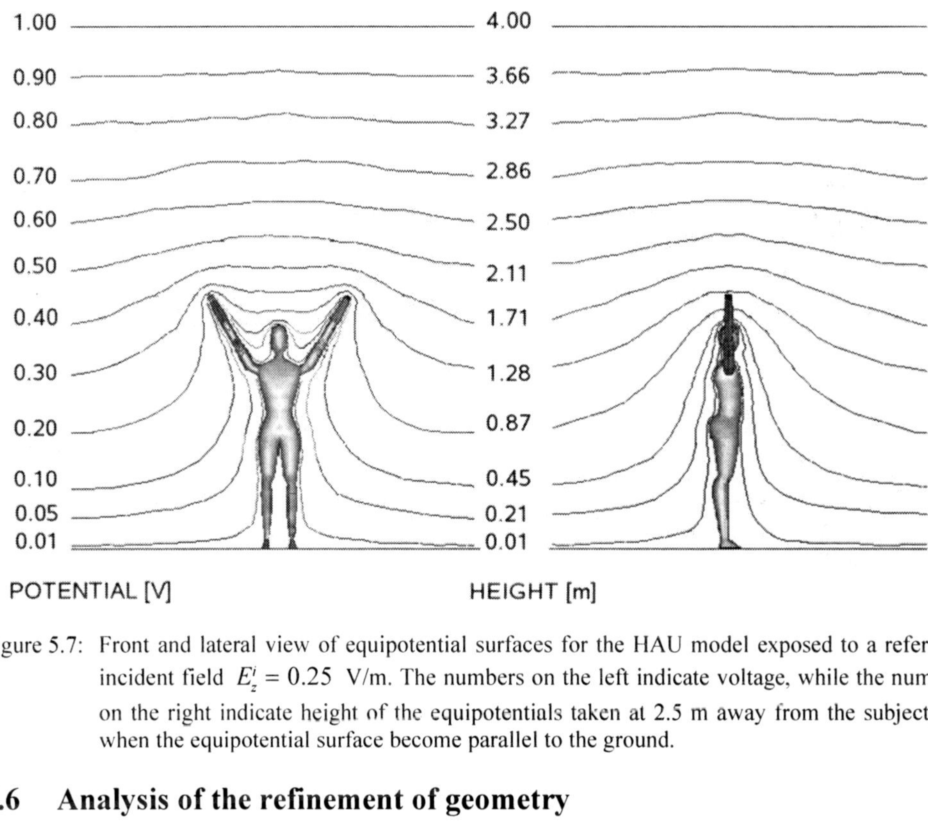

Figure 5.7: Front and lateral view of equipotential surfaces for the HAU model exposed to a reference incident field E_z^i = 0.25 V/m. The numbers on the left indicate voltage, while the numbers on the right indicate height of the equipotentials taken at 2.5 m away from the subject, i.e. when the equipotential surface become parallel to the ground.

5.6 Analysis of the refinement of geometry

One of the most evident physical differences that arise in human anatomy definition is the difference on the geometry of one subject in relation to another. In order to clarify the influence of the geometry definition on the induced electric field and current density, simulations for different models have been performed and are summarised in the following paragraphs.

5.6.1 Influence of the cross-sectional area

In order to demonstrate the influence of the geometry on the induced current density in the human bodies, a comparison between a cylindrical and an anatomical representation of the body is introduced in this section. The axial induced current density (j_z) has been calculated along the longitudinal axis $\hat{z}$ of the human body for the cylindrical CYL model as well as for the HNA model. Results corresponding to an incident field of 10 kV/m are shown in Figure 5.8. The observation line corresponds to the line connecting points A and B in Figure 5.3(a), where z varies between 1.75 and 0.85 m. Below $z = 0.85$ m, the observation line passes through the centre of one leg.

In the CYL model, a gradual rise in the current density is measured from head to feet as z decreases from 1.75 to 0 m. This can be explained considering that the current flowing across a section normal to the applied field depends on the sum of the surface charge on the body above that section. In fact, the HNA model shows the same behaviour between head and feet. However, a decrease followed by a rise in the cross-sectional area causes a rise in the current density followed by a fall. If the change in the cross-sectional area is significant, it is possible to find lower currents at the shoulder's height ($z = 1.4$ m) than those corresponding to the neck ($z = 1.5$ m).

In the HNA model four well-identified peaks appear at the levels of the neck, waist, knee and ankle. Therefore, the results indicate that an over-simplified representation of the human body such as the cylindrical or ellipsoidal models are unable to capture the effect of high current densities in regions of reduced cross section. Peak values are summarised in Table 5.4. Results obtained are comparable with those obtained by different methods and presented in earlier publications such as references [19, 25, 109].

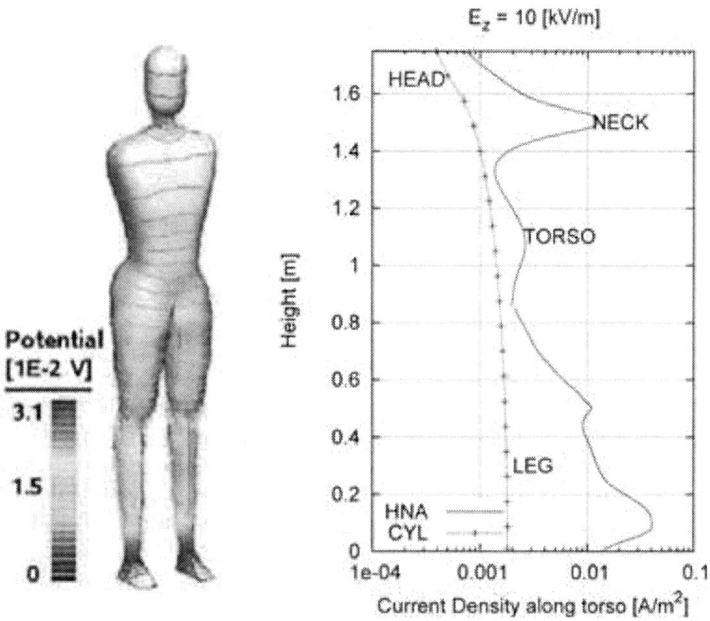

Figure 5.8: Axial component of the induced current density along the human body for the models CYL and HNA.

Table 5.4: Peak values of axial current density for HNA and CYL models.

Height	j_{zHNA} [mA/m^2]	j_{zCYL} [mA/m^2]
Neck	12.1	0.9
Knee	11	1.6
Ankle	40	2

5.6.2 Inclusion of arms

In order to analyse the influence of the inclusion of arms in the model as well as the variation on the orientation of the arms in relation with the incident field, a comparison between models with arms positioned on sides, arms raised at different angles and without the inclusion of arms has been considered (HAD, HAO, HAU and HNA models have been introduced in Section 5.3).

The axial current density (j_z) flowing to ground as well as the axial current along the arms have been calculated for all the models mentioned above.

5.6.2.1 Current density along the head and torso

Figure 5.9 shows the comparison of the axial current distribution j_z^1 along a vertical line in $\hat{z}$ direction that passes through the centre of the head and torso. The comparison is done between the models HAU, HAO, HAD and HNA corresponding to the human body with raised arms, horizontally elevated, arms down on the sides and no arms at all, respectively. The results correspond to an incident field of 10 kV/m. In the region between $z = 0.85$ and $z = 1.4$ m (torso), it can be seen that the current density increases as the arms are raised according to reference [105]. For the HAO and HAU models, the effect of the bigger area exposed to a normal field in the case of the HAO model competes with the effect that takes place in the case of the HAU model, in which a smaller area is exposed to a higher intensity field. The results show that HAU model gives the highest total current density. Table 5.5 shows the corresponding peak values of current density for the different models, which are typically found in the neck and waist. Along the torso, the smallest values are reached in the chest and are close to 2 mA/m^2 for all the models. Finally, in case of the peak corresponding to the neck, the general behaviour of the current density is reversed and the current decreases as the arms are raised.

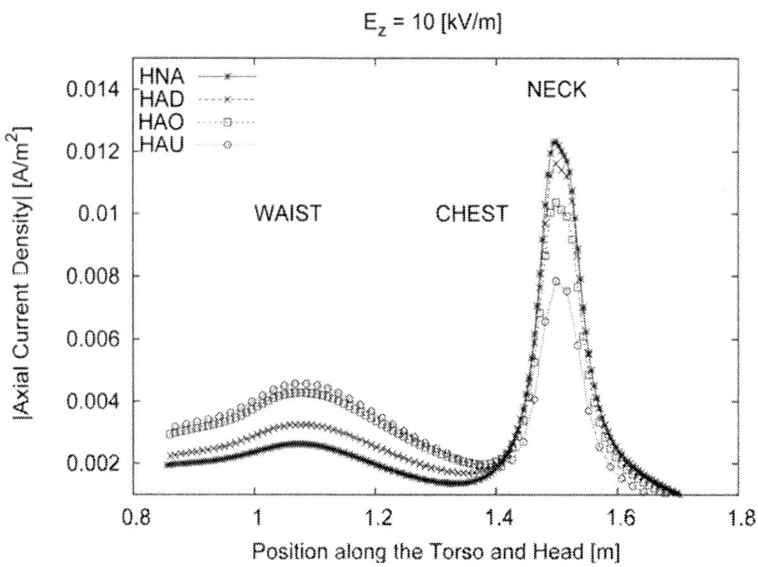

Figure 5.9: Distribution of axial current density along the torso and head in function of the height for the HAU, HAO, HAD and HNA models. The observation line corresponds to the line connecting points A and B in Figure 5.3(a).

Table 5.5: Peak of axial current density.

j_z [mA/m^2]	Neck	Waist	Knee	Ankle
HNA	12.1	2.5	11	40
HAD	11.8	3.1	12	43
HAO	10.2	4	18	60
HAU	8	4.3	18	60

5.6.2.2 Current density along the arms

Figure 5.10 shows the absolute value of the axial current density, $|\mathbf{j}\cdot\hat{s}|$, along the arm coordinate (s), where $\hat{s}$ is the longitudinal axis of the arm, for all the models. The results correspond to an incident field of 10 kV/m. In each model, the calculation line passes through the centre of the arm. In the grounded model of the human body, **j** is mainly oriented parallel to the longitudinal axis of the limbs. It can be noticed as well that the current density reaches the highest values, in case of the HAO model, in accordance to the larger area exposed to the normal field. The smallest values are found in the case of HAD model, as it can be expected due to the small area exposed in conjunction with the lower intensity field. The absolute value in this case is smaller than 3 mA/m^2, so it can be expected that almost all the current goes through the body. In accordance with the definition of the geometry of the arm, the cross section presents more variations in case of the HAO model. For the HAU model, the variations of the cross section are less significant and for the HAD model they are even smoother. This explains the presence of more peaks in case of the HAO model, for the regions corresponding to the elbow and at a distance of 17 cm from the chest, after the biceps. Moreover, a local minimum is seen in the zone of the biceps where the cross-sectional area reaches a maximum. For the HAD model, the practically constant cross-sectional area is reflected in the values obtained for the related current density. Details of the geometry of the arms are given in Figure 5.11.

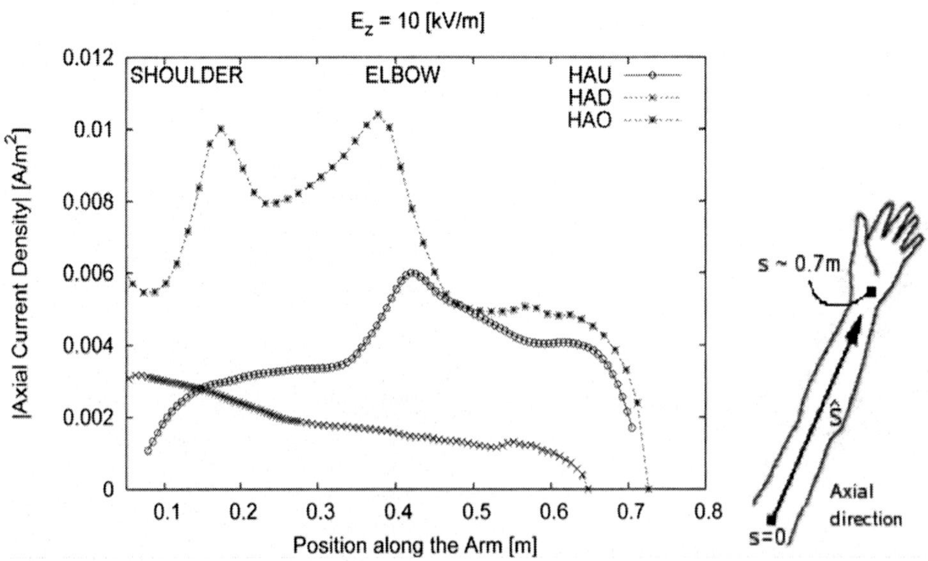

Figure 5.10: Absolute value of axial current density along arms $|\mathbf{j}\cdot\hat{s}|$ in function of the distance along the arm s for the HAU, HAO and HAD models.

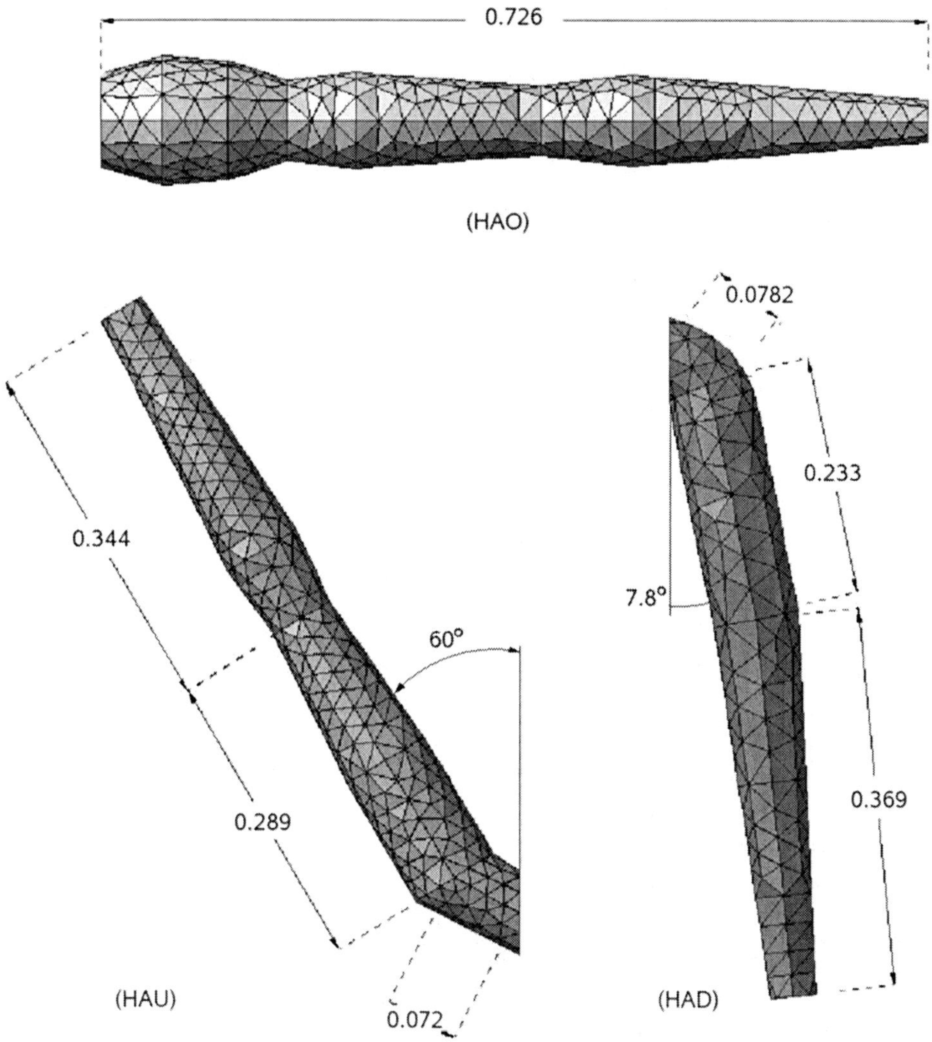

Figure 5.11: Geometry of the arms in HAU, HAO and HAD models.

5.6.2.3 Current density along the legs

Figure 5.12 compares the absolute values of the axial current distribution (i.e. the component of **j** parallel to the longitudinal axis of the leg) along a line that passes through the centre of the leg for the HNA, HAD, HAO and HAU models, for an incident field of 10 kV/m. All of them show the presence of two well-identified peaks corresponding to the reduction in the cross-sectional area at the height of the ankle and knee. The maximum values of current density at the height of the ankle are typically of 60 mA/m^2 for the HAU and HAO models and close to 50 mA/m^2 for the HAD and HNA models, as it has been assigned in Table 5.5. At the knee, all models have current density values of the order of 20 mA/m^2 or even lower.

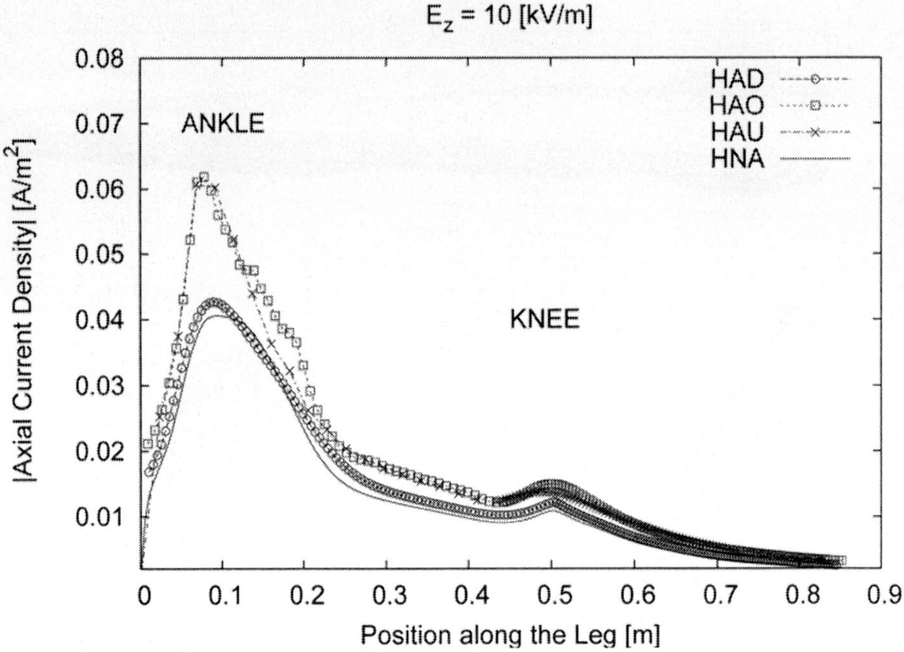

Figure 5.12: Axial current density along the legs in function of the lenght for the HAU, HAO, HAD and HNA models.

Finally, it can be concluded that the total current density along the legs has the same behaviour as along the torso, reaching its maximum at the ankle. The ankles, knees and neck appeared to be the most vulnerable regions of the body within the given circumstances.

5.6.3 Inclusion of organs

In order to estimate the influence of the inclusion of organs on the induced current density, the response of the HIO model, which includes some relevant internal organs such as brain, eyes, heart and intestine; and the homogeneous HNA model has been compared. Figure 5.13 shows the results for the current density measured along the torso with an incident field of 10 kV/m. The observation line passes through the centre of the body and corresponds to the line connecting points A and B in Figure 5.3. The conductivity values for the different organs are summarised in Table 5.6. Three sets of conductivity values have been included in the table, namely SETA, SETG and SETD. The first one, SETA dataset has been used in this example. For the embedding medium, the conductivity is ascribed as the conductivity of muscle. As can be noticed for SETA dataset, the conductivity of the internal organs is relatively lower than the conductivity of the medium in which the organs are embedded, thus yielding some local depressions of current density observed between 0.8 m and 1.3 m. The observation line, which extends from $(x, y, z) = 0, 0, 0.82$ to $(x, y, z) = 0, 0, 1.75$, interferes with the intestine between $z = 0.93$ m and $z = 1.07$ m (points A and B, respectively), hence the first depression observed in the figure. Then, the current rapidly increases in the subsequent region of higher conductivity until it reaches the liver at point C which causes another depression between 1.15 m and 1.2 m. Although the heart does not interfere with the observation line, its presence can be sensed near $z = 1.28$ m (point C), where it is at its minimum distance of nearly 2 cm. Therefore, due to its lower conductivity, the heart will cause a local maximum in the adjacent region considered as a saline solution (point D). Furthermore, in this model the value of axial current density computed at the centre of the heart is given by the following equation:

$$j_z^{(\text{heart})} = \alpha E_z, \tag{5.3}$$

where $\alpha = (4.4 \pm 0.1) \times 10^{-8}$ A/V/m and E_z is the vertical electric field at ground level measured without the human body (i.e. 0.4 mA/m^2 underneath a 10 kV/m power line). The peak at point E is correlated to the reduction of the cross section in the neck and its value is insensitive to variations on the location and conductivities of the internal organs. Then, the current density decreases as the exposed cross section increases from the neck to the centre of the head. Finally, the last depression is found between points E and G due to the lower conductivity of the brain. As observed in Figure 5.13, the HNA model gives an envelope of the HIO.

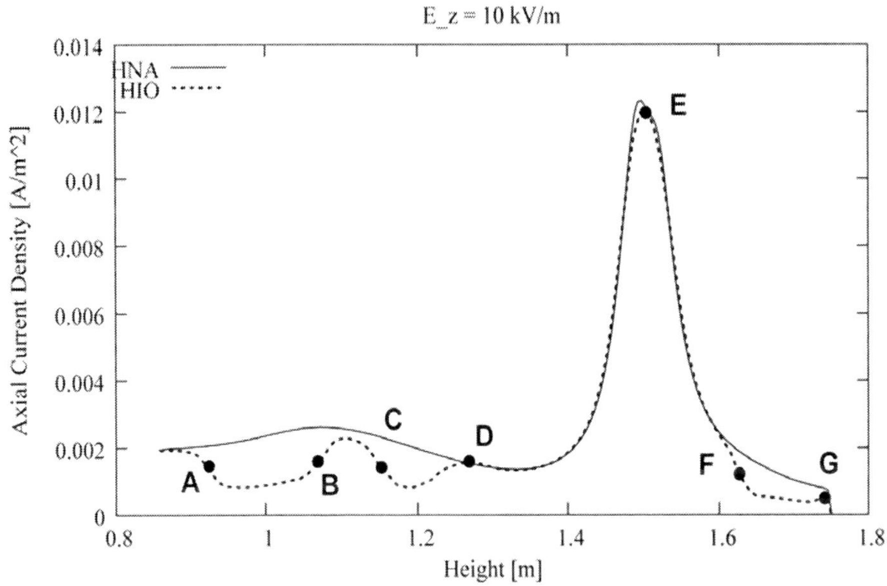

Figure 5.13: Axial current density along the torso and head in function of the height for the HIO and HNA models.

Table 5.6: Selected tissue conductivities in S/m at 60 Hz.

Tissue	SETA	σ_t/σ_m	SETG	σ_t/σ_m	SETD
Embedding tissue	0.50	1.00	0.22	1.00	0.44
Heart	0.11	0.22	0.08	0.36	0.16
Brain	0.12	0.24	0.04	0.18	0.08
Eye	0.11	0.22	1.0	4.55	2.0
Liver	0.13	0.26	0.07	0.32	0.14
Intestine	0.16	0.32	1.15	5.27	2.30

SETA dataset has been extracted from the work of Gandhi [25], while SETG dataset from Gabriel et al. [66]. The ratio between tissue conductivity and the embedding medium (σ_t/σ_m) is included.

5.7 Analysis of variations on conductivity

In order to analyse the influence of tissue conductivity on the induced electric field and current density within the body, different experiments have been conducted.

5.7.1 Variations on conductivity in the homogeneous representation

Figure 5.14(a–f) shows the comparison for current density and electric field obtained when different tissue conductivities are assigned to the body in the homogeneous representation HNA. Three different values of conductivity σ = 0.01, 0.3 and 5 S/m are chosen to be compared with standard value σ = 0.5 S/m.

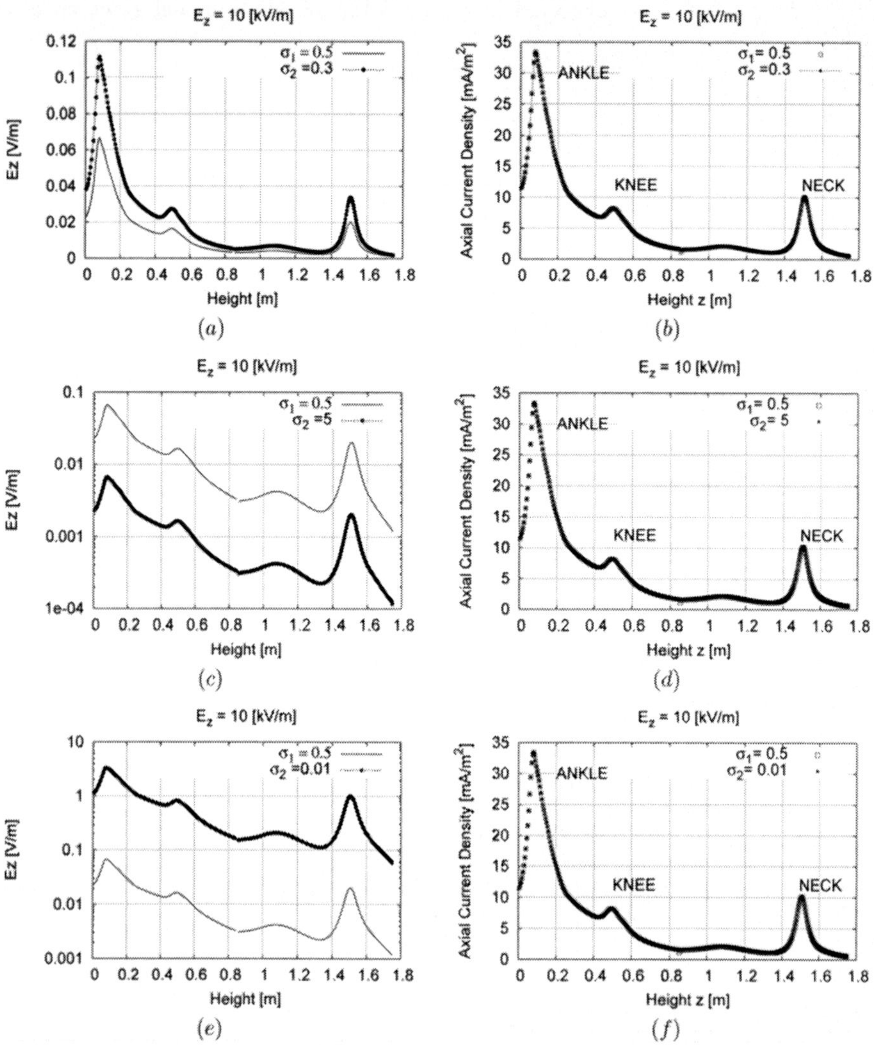

Figure 5.14: Axial current density and electric field along the centre of the torso and legs for the HNA model with conductivities σ_1 and σ_2 in [S/m].

As revealed in Figure 5.14(b, d and f) the current density remains the same in all the cases. In fact, this result is expected in the homogeneous representation due to the presence of the air, which can be thought as a conductor with apparent conductivity σ_{ap} which at 60 Hz is equal to:

$$\sigma_{ap} = \omega\varepsilon_0 = 3.8410^{-9}\,\text{S/m}. \tag{5.4}$$

Alternatively, it can be assigned a resistivity of the order of 10^9 Ω/m and the whole system can be represented as a very large resistor in series with another resistor representing the tissue with resistivity ranging approximately between 2 and 3 Ω/m. Therefore, a small variation in the conductivity of the homogeneous tissue does not affect the current density which is dominated by the air material properties.

However, the variation in the induced electric field is related to the variation in the conductivity. As can be seen, when comparing the conductivities 0.5 and 0.3 S/m in Figure 5.14(a), for the peaks at the ankle and waist the electric field decreases by 60% for a decrease of 58% in the conductivities. For the peak at the neck, the decrease in the electric field is of 55%.

Also, in case (e) (Figure 5.14(e)), which compares conductivities of 0.5 and 0.01 S/m, a decrease factor of 50 in the ratio of conductivities is translated into a decrease in the induced electric field by the same factor.

Finally, in case (c) where the conductivity increases by a factor of 10, the induced electric field increases, as expected, by the same factor.

5.7.2 Variations of conductivity in the heterogeneous representation

In this section, the induced current density is calculated for different conductivity distributions, namely SETA, SETG and SETD, in the heterogeneous representation HIO. The different conductivity distributions are summarised in Table 5.6.

Data from SETA and SETG sets has been extracted from literature, while data from SETD dataset was obtained by multiplying all the conductivity values in SETG dataset by a factor of 2.

SETG dataset has been extracted from Gabriel et al. [67]. It is commonly used by many researchers and has been derived, as described in Chapter 3, by integrating tissue conductivity values into NORMAN model. SETA dataset is commonly used in the work of Gandhi [25]. As can be seen in the table, SETG dataset is similar to SETA dataset in some aspects. Although the conductivity used for the embedding medium is lower in the case of SETG, the ratio of variation between the conductivity of the medium and the conductivity of tissue is practically the same in the case of heart, brain and liver. In contrast, the difference between both sets is evident in the case of the eyes and intestine in which the conductivities for SETG, unlike what happens in SETA, are significantly higher than the conductivity of the surrounding medium.

5.7.2.1 Comparison between different conductivity distributions

Figure 5.15 shows the comparison of current density calculated along a vertical line in z direction that passes through the centre of the head and torso for the three conductivity distributions SETA, SETG and SETD, as well as for the homogeneous representation HNA labelled as SETH. The incident field is 10 kV/m. In this example, SETH conductivity is 0.5 S/m. However, as has been discussed in the previous section, any value assigned to the conductivity in the homogeneous representation will give the same values of induced current density. As can be seen in Figure 5.15, in all the cases the local minimums are associated with the organs in which conductivities are lower than the conductivity of the medium such as brain, heart and liver. Despite the fact that the calculation line does not pass through the heart, in all cases its presence is sensed with a local maximum as discussed in Section 5.6.3. The intestine has higher conductivity than the medium in the case of SETG and SETD distributions and was accompanied with an increase in the current density, compared with SETA dataset in which the conductivity of the liver is also lower than the conductivity of the surrounding medium. Except for the intestine, the overall behaviour is very similar for the three distributions and the homogeneous curve still acts as an envelope for the SETG and SETD datasets. As expected, it is inferred from the results that as long as the ratio between the conductivity of the surrounding medium and the considered tissue is small, the general behaviour of the current density will be very similar to the behaviour obtained with the homogeneous representation, whereas the highest value of current density has been obtained in the case of intestine and eyes, in which the ratios are 5.27 and 4.55, respectively.

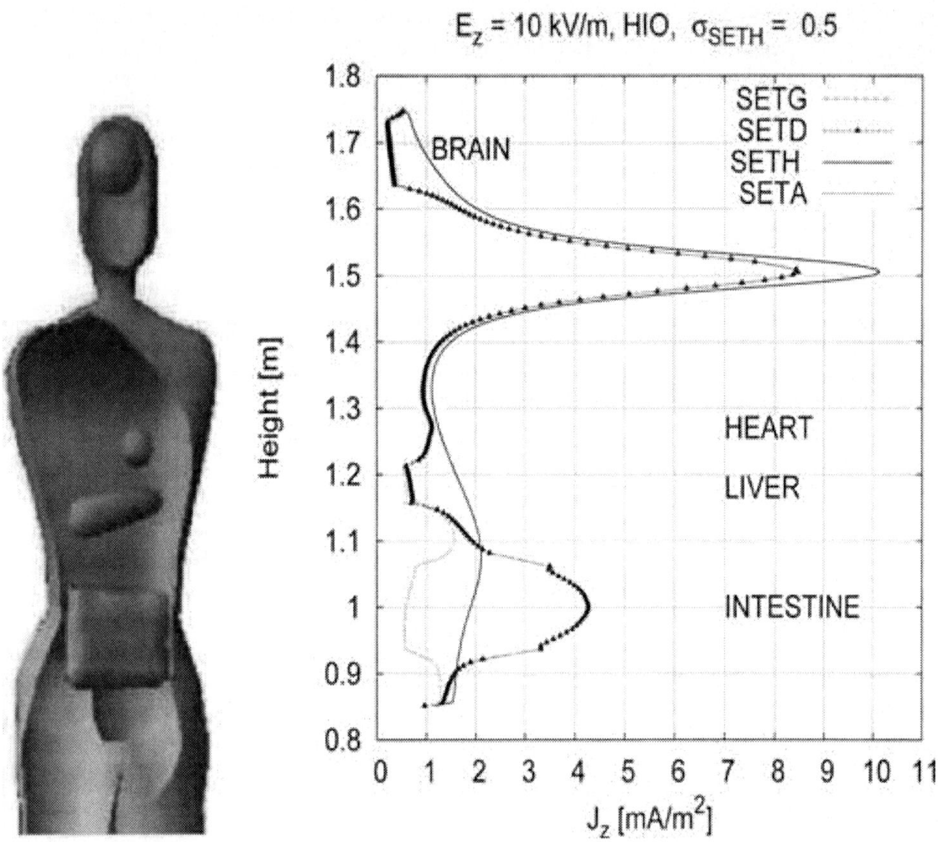

Figure 5.15: Axial current density along the centre of the torso and head for the HIO model with different sets of conductivities. For the homogeneous model the conductivity is set to 0.5 S/m.

Finally, it is worth noticing that when the whole set is multiplied by the same factor and the ratio σ_t/σ_m keeps the same for both sets, as in the case of SETG and SETD, the same values of current density are obtained for both datasets as expected.

The induced electric field calculated in the vertical direction z along a line that passes through the centre of the head and torso for the different sets of conductivities SETA, SETD, SETG is shown in Figures 5.16 and 5.17. Additionally, as a reference, a homogeneous representation HNA has been included, labelled as SETH1 and SETH2 with conductivities of 0.5 and 0.22 S/m, respectively. As seen, the maximum value of the electric field occurs at the neck for all the datasets, ranging between 17 mV/m in case of SETA dataset and 37 mV/m for SETG dataset. The different conductivities of the organs yield to depressions and peaks as reasoned previously in the case of the current density, but conversely, i.e. in regions where the conductivity is lower than the surrounding medium such as brain and liver, the induced electric field experiences an increase, whether in regions where the conductivity of the organ is higher than the surrounding medium, like intestine in the case of SETG and SETD the field decreases. From the comparison in Figure 5.16, it can be noticed that for SETG the values obtained are very similar than those obtained for the homogeneous representation (SETH2). However for SETD distribution, the field decreases by a factor 1/2 for all the organs, as expected. The lowest values of induced electric field are reached in the case of SETA distribution.

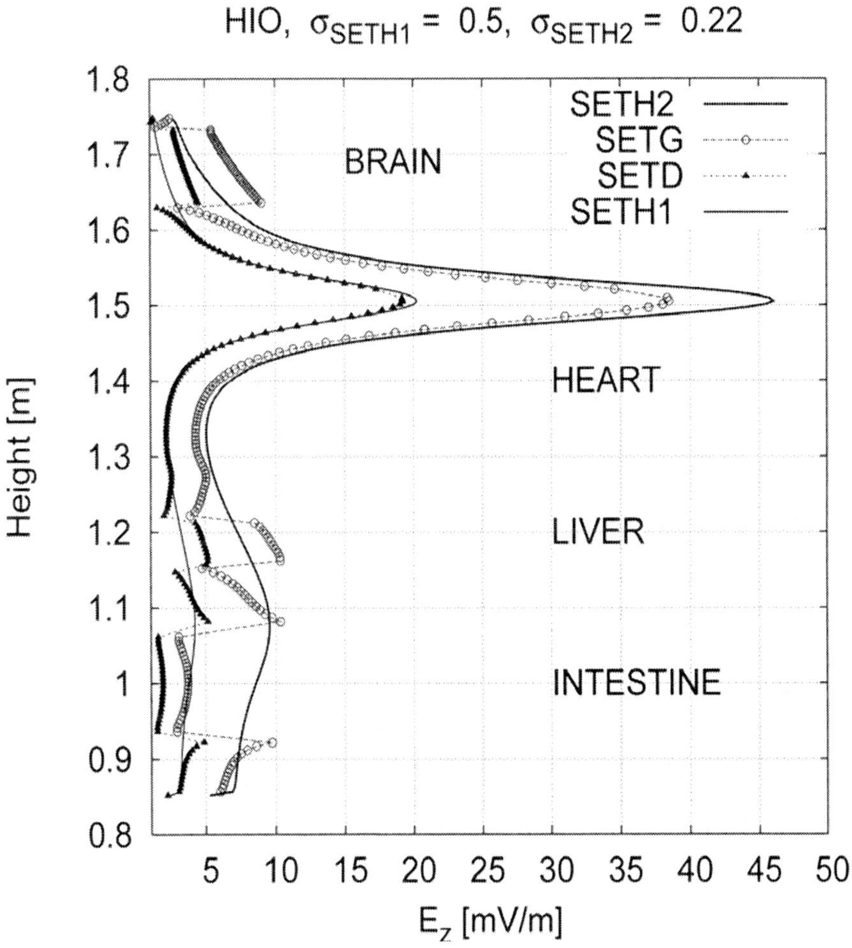

Figure 5.16: Vertical induced electric field in mV/m calculated along the centre of the torso and head for the HIO model for SETG and SETD conductivity distributions. A homogeneous representation has been included, with conductivities of 0.5 and 0.2 S/m labelled as SETH1 and SETH2, respectively.

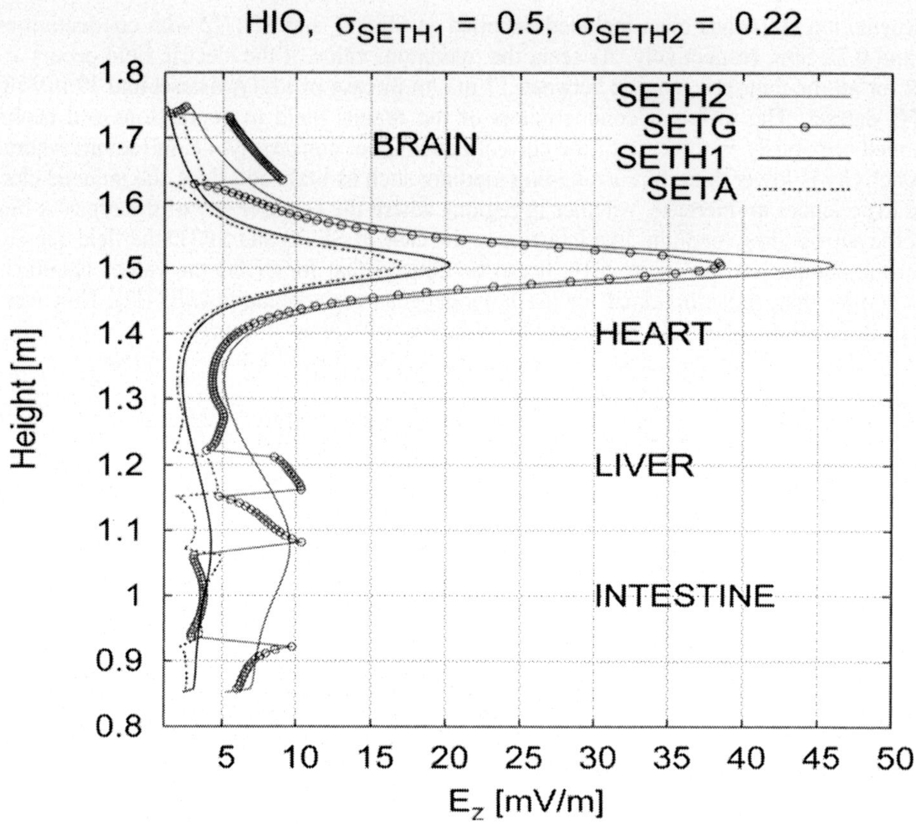

Figure 5.17: Vertical induced electric field in mV/m calculated along the centre of the torso and head for the HIO model for SETG and SETA conductivity distributions. A homogeneous representation has been included, with conductivities of 0.5 and 0.2 S/m labelled as SETH1 and SETH2, respectively.

5.7.2.2 Conductivity of the embedding medium

In order to analyse the response of the induced current density to variations in the conductivity assigned to the surrounding medium, the following examples have been studied. From SETG dataset, a series of different sets have been generated by modifying only the conductivity of the embedding medium. To proceed with the comparison, the conductivities of the medium have been prescribed as follows: 0.05, 0.5 and 2.20 S/m and will be referred as G-0.05, G-0.50 and G-2.20, respectively. The comparison of the current density and electric field obtained with the former distributions and SETG dataset is shown in Figure 5.18 for an incident field of 10 kV/m. The calculation line, in $\hat{z}$ direction, passes through the centre of the head and torso.

Table 5.7 illustrates the ratios of conductivities between the correspondent tissue and the medium σ_m/σ_t for each dataset. For SETG distribution, the conductivity values of the organs are similar in the case of the heart, liver and brain, ranging between 0.04 and 0.08 S/m, whereas the values for the intestine and eyes are also similar but significantly higher than in the previous organs, being 1.15 and 1 S/m, respectively.

Table 5.7: Ratios σ_t/σ_m for SETG, G-0.05, G-0.50 and G-2.20 datasets.

Tissue	σ_{SETG}	$\sigma_t/0.05$	$\sigma_t/0.22$	$\sigma_t/0.5$	$\sigma_t/2.2$
Brain	0.04	0.8	0.18	0.08	0.02
Heart	0.08	1.60	0.36	0.16	0.04
Liver	0.07	1.40	0.32	0.14	0.03
Intestine	1.15	23.0	5.27	2.30	0.53
Eye	1.0	20.0	4.55	2.00	0.46

In case of the G-0.05 distribution, the ratio σ_t/σ_m is higher than 1 for the heart and liver and lower than 1 for the brain, but still close to 1 for the three of them. Thus, this will be reflected in the current density flowing through them, in which practically the curve is very similar to the homogeneous curve from z = 1.75 to 1.10 m. For the brain, it experiences a decrease by the same factor than the ratio of conductivities ($1 - \sigma_t/\sigma_m$), i.e. a decrease of 20% respect to the current density in the homogeneous case. In case of the liver, the ratio of conductivities is higher than 1, therefore an increase in current density is expected. For heart, the ratio is 1.6, thus yielding an increment of 60% which will produce an increment in the current density flowing through the heart and consequently this is sensed in the neighbourhood and reflected as a decrease in the current density which can be seen in Figure 5.18(a).

In comparison with SETG dataset, G-0.05 produce also similar current densities flowing along the head and chest (from z = 1.75 to 1.10 m), with small differences in the organs that can be explained comparing the variation relative to the embedding medium of the conductivity of the correspondent organ. For instance, for brain the conductivity in SETG is 81% lower than the conductivity of the embedding medium, thus yielding a decrease of the same amount with respect to the homogeneous representation. Regarding the peak that occurs at the height corresponding to the neck at z = 1.49 m, both conductivity distributions SETG and G-0.05 reach the same value of 8.3 mA/m, which is lower than the one reached in the homogeneous representation. For the intestine, the ratio between σ_t/σ_m is 5.27 in the case of SETG and 23 in the case of G-0.05, thus yielding to a significant increase in the current density proportional to these differences.

The comparison between G-0.5 and SETG distributions is shown in Figure 5.18(c). G-0.5 represents a dataset very similar to SETG dataset in the sense that as the conductivity of the medium is 0.5, the inequalities between organs and medium are maintained in the same way than that in SETG. As discussed earlier, the depressions corresponding to the brain, heart and liver, as well as the peak corresponding to the intestine are reproduced by both models. However, in this case, G-0.5, the depressions are deeper than in SETG dataset, because the difference between conductivities is bigger. Similar to the former comparison between G-0.05 and SETG for the peak at the neck, both conductivity distributions G-0.5 and SETG give very similar values.

Finally, the comparison between G-2.20 and SETG datasets is shown in Figure 5.18(e). The conductivity of the surrounding medium is higher than the conductivity of all the organs thus yielding depressions for all of them. Because the difference of conductivity between the surrounding medium and brain and liver is higher, the depressions are more pronounced in this case. For the intestine, the difference between conductivities is smaller thus yielding a depression proportional to this difference. Similarly, as the previous examples, at the neck the current density remains the same for SETG and G-2.20.

It is worth mentioning that the current density remains the same for all the distributions in the regions corresponding to the embedding medium, independently of the conductivities of the different organs and its relation with the conductivity of the embedding medium.

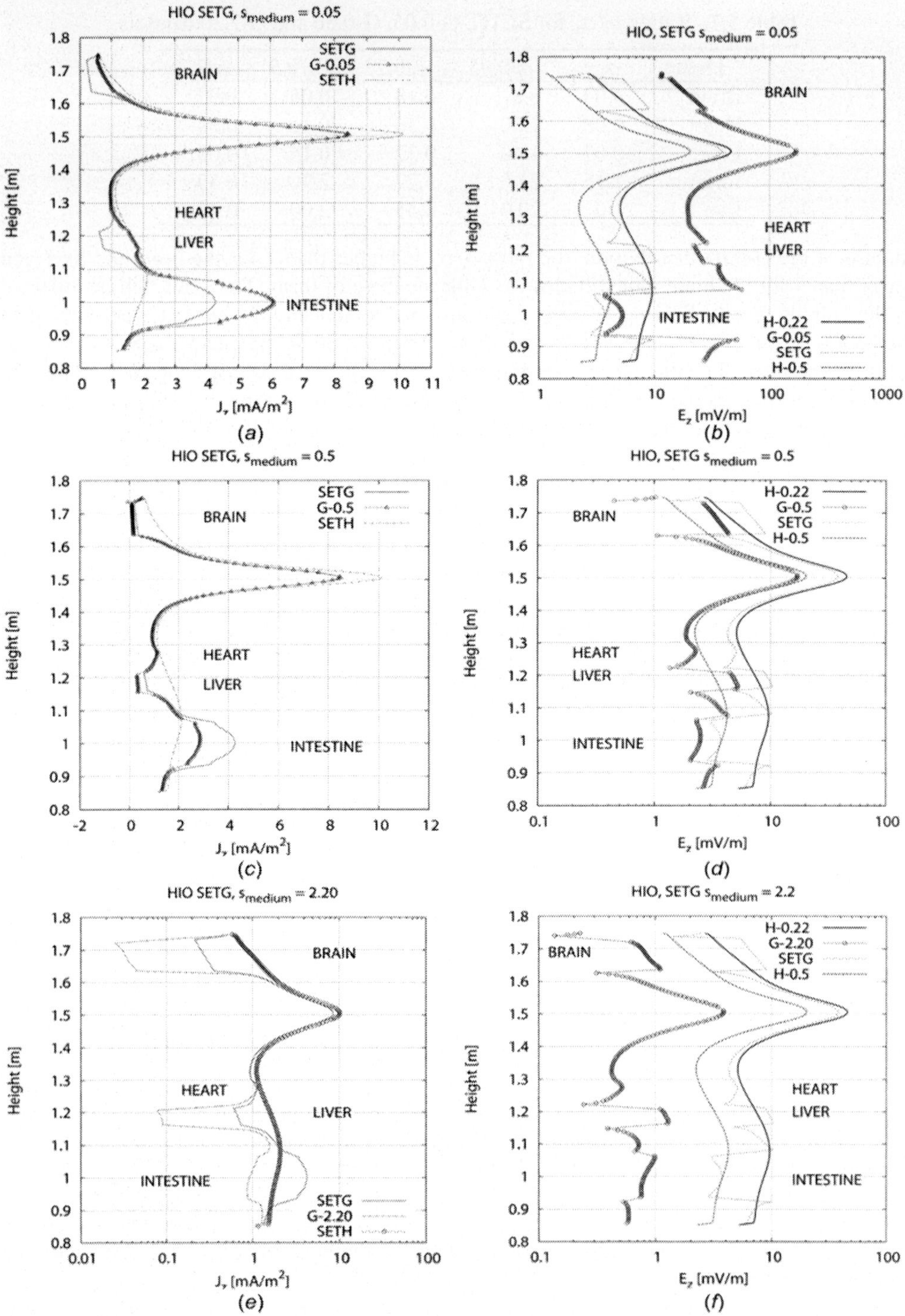

Figure 5.18: The comparison of the current density and electric field obtained with the former distributions and SETG dataset.

5.7.2.3 Normal component of electric field E_n on the skin

Figure 5.19(a) shows the normal field along the skin for the SETG and SETA datasets. The difference between the normal components of the electric field for both conductivity distributions is plotted in (b).

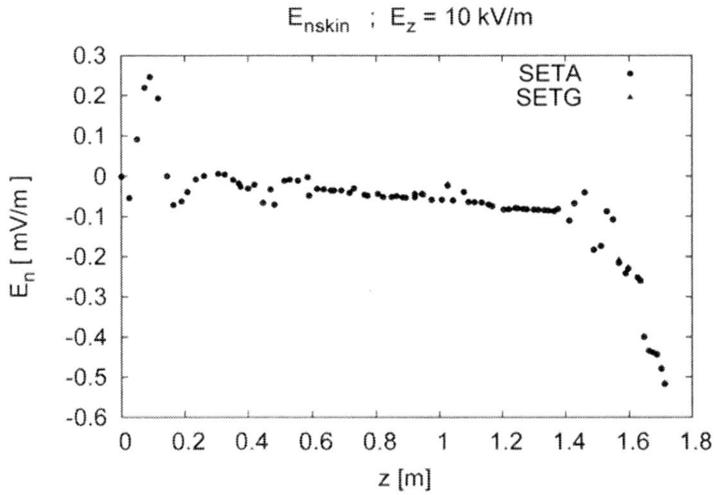

(a)

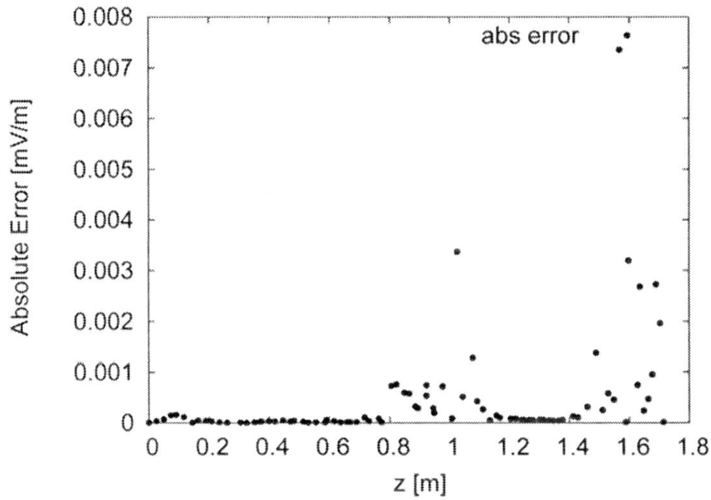

(b)

Figure 5.19: (a) Normal electric field at the external surface (skin) of the body for SETG and SETA distributions. (b) Error between the normal electric field of the two models.

This result demonstrates that the normal field induced on the surface of the body does not depend on the conductivity distribution of the internal (embedded) organs. In fact, it is observed that one of the most influential factors is the external geometry of the body. Therefore, the conductivity distribution inside the body does not affect the field on the surface representing the body.

5.8 Summary

The results obtained in this chapter show that the current density produced in the human body exposed to an incident electric field parallel to the length of the body, depends almost entirely on the size of the cross-sectional area normally exposed. From the analysis of the refinement of geometry, it can be summarised that the peak values appear in the neck, knees and ankles, and the localisation of these peaks shown to be insensitive to variations on the position of the arms. The total current density along the torso and legs is significantly increased as the arms are raised. Although in the head and neck, this behaviour is reverted, and the neck is protected as the arms are raised, due to the expected screening effect. In this sense, the brain would as well be protected as the arms are raised. Along the chest, the cross-sectional area normally exposed reaches its maximum. Consequently, this represents a natural protection for the heart. Finally, it is worth mentioning that the model without arms is useful to determine the localisation of the peaks and orders of average values of current densities, but fails to predict the 33% increase in the cases with arms raised for the peak values in the ankle and knee, as well as the significant decrease of 33% in the neck and head. From the sensibility analysis for the conductivity, it can be summarised that the influence of the internal distribution on the current density flowing through the body is important in the case where the ratio between conductivities of the different tissues considered is big, whereas as long as the ratio between the conductivity of the surrounding medium and the considered tissue is small, the homogeneous representation represents a good approximation of the general behaviour of the current density and induced electric field, which are dominated by the variations on the geometry. Moreover, if the conductivity of a particular tissue is lower than the conductivity of the medium, this is translated into a depression in the current density flowing through that tissue and a local maximum in the current density flowing through the medium in the proximity of the tissue.

It has been verified that due to the highly resistive properties of air in homogeneous representation, the variation in conductivity does not affect the current density flowing in the interior of the body.

It has been demonstrated that the normal field induced on the surface of the body does not depend on the conductivity distribution of the internal (embedded) organs.

Results can be compared with the basic restrictions established in reference [2]. As a reference, the ICNIRP establishes a maximum value of 10 mA/m^2, in case of exposure to ELF fields of frequency between 4 Hz and 1 kHz, for head and trunk in the working population and 2 mA/m^2 for general public. The results found in this work, excluding the neck, are below the limit for working population, however proximity to the radiation source may easily increase this value. Results obtained for current density are in good agreement with earlier publications by Gandhi et al. (1992), King (2004) [19, 24, 25, 105, 110].

Note

1 In this case **j** in the torso is mostly oriented parallel to the vertical direction, i.e. $|\mathbf{j}\cdot\hat{z}| \sim |\mathbf{j}|$.

6

Exposure in power substations rooms

6.1 Introduction

Substation transformers are designed for a wide range of commercial, industrial and utility applications. The usual activities of a power substation operator involve touching of control units, connecting and disconnecting switches as well as other grounded metallic objects exposed to high electrical fields. As a result, when a person is either in the proximity of or in contact with conductive surfaces at different potentials, induced and contact currents may flow throughout the different tissues. Pre-contact spark discharge currents may also occur. This chapter deals with a realistic parametric model of the grounded human body standing inside a power substation room, in order to estimate the current density along the body for different possible exposure scenarios in a substation room. Section 6.2 shows the results obtained for a 3D model representing the human body located in the interior of a substation transformer under different situations of exposure. Section 6.3 analyses the exposure of a worker in a power substation room in terms of induced currents and fields in the proximity of panels at fixed voltages.

6.2 Induced currents in the human body inside a power substation room

In this example, a grounded human body is assumed to be located in the vicinity of a transformer substation. Figure 6.1 shows the integration domain, which consists of a cylinder of 2 m in height and 0.6 m diameter. The electric field generated in the vicinity of substations vary appreciably depending on the geometry, the design, etc. According to reference [111], an electric field of 380 V/m applied as boundary condition in the near field of the human body has been considered as a reasonable representation of typical human exposure conditions in a substation room. The induced current in different situations for the HNA model of the body is analysed. The examples studied include three scenarios: the first case considers the human body exposed to a vertical field of 380 V/m. This has been achieved by imposing the following boundary conditions: $E_n = 0$ in the lateral surface of the cylinder and $\varphi = 760$ V applied to the top surface of the cylinder. In the second case, the vertical component of the electric field is null, but the normal component is equal to 380 V/m. These conditions were achieved by imposing $\varphi = 0$ to the top surface of the cylinder, and normal electric field $E_n = 380$ V/m to the lateral surface of the cylinder. In the third case, both the components, vertical and normal ones are equal to 380 V/m. The imposed boundary conditions were $\varphi = 760$ V/m to the top surface and $E_n = 380$ V/m to the lateral surface.

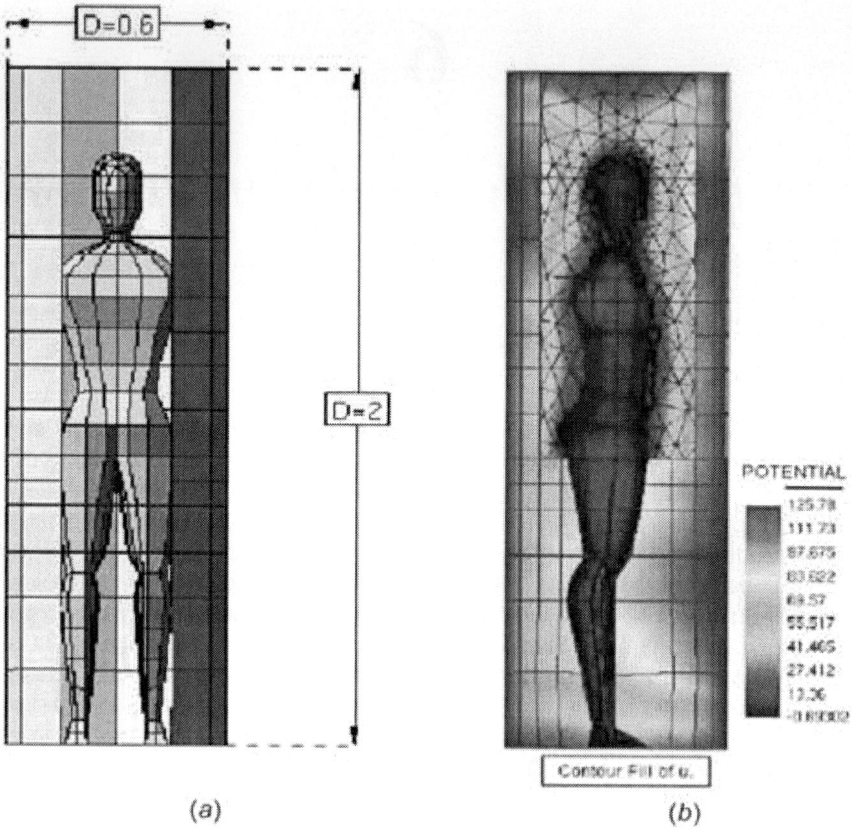

Figure 6.1: (a) Integration domain for the substation. (b) Equipotential 380 V/m.

In the three examples, the bottom surface of the cylinder has been kept grounded, i.e. $\varphi = 0$. The conditions for the three different scenarios has been summarised in Table 6.1.

Table 6.1: Different exposure scenarios boundary conditions.

	Vertical incident field	Boundary conditions
Scenario A	$E_z = 380$ V/m	$E_n = 0$ in the lateral surface of the cylinder
	$E_n = 0$	$\varphi = 760$ V on the top surface of the cylinder
	Horizontal incident field	Boundary conditions
Scenario B	$E_n = 380$ V/m	$\varphi = 0$ on the top surface of the cylinder
	$E_z = 0$	$E_n = 380$ V/m on the lateral surface of the cylinder
	Incident field	Boundary conditions
Scenario C	$E_n = 380$ V/m	$\varphi = 760$ V/m on the top surface
	$E_z = 380$ V/m	$E_n = 380$ V/m on the lateral surface

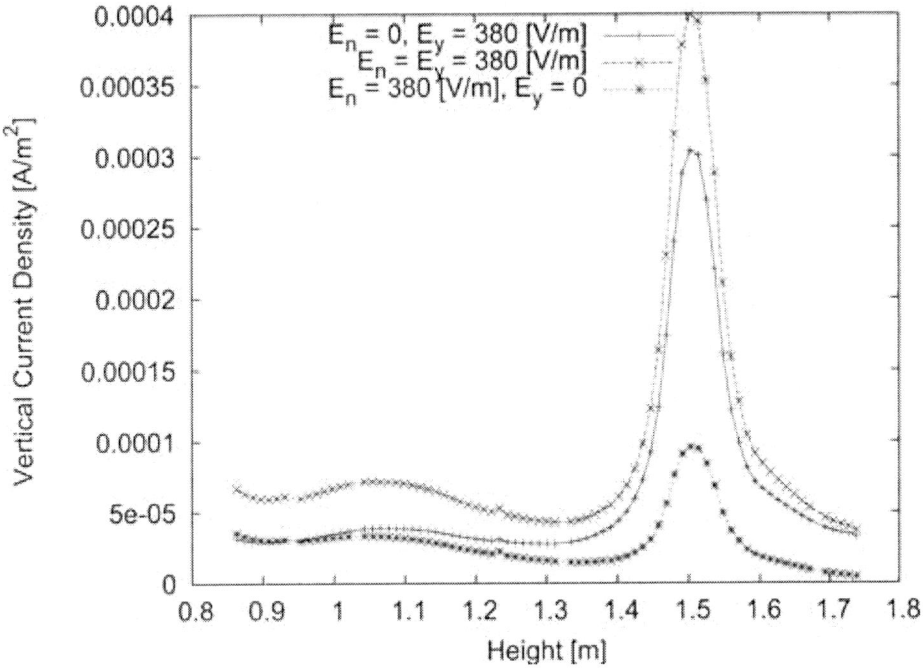

Figure 6.2: Vertical current density along the torso and head.

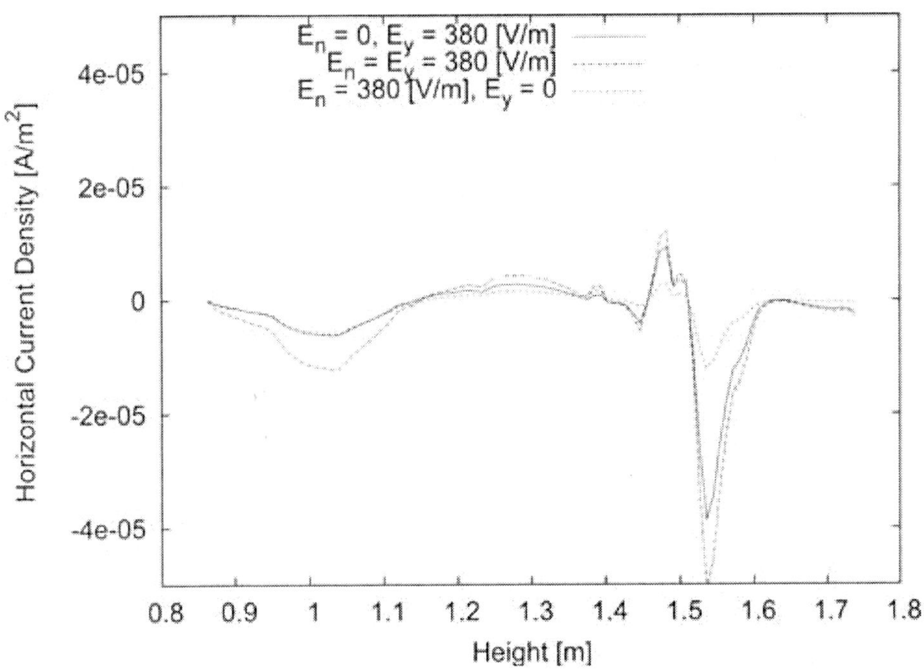

Figure 6.3: Normal current density along the torso and head.

The results are shown in Figure 6.2, where the vertical component of the current density for different scenarios is plotted along the torso and head. It reflects the same general behaviour as the previous case of power-lines, showing peaks at the height corresponding to the waist and neck. The normal component of the current density is negligible in these cases as seen in Figure 6.3. In these examples the number of elements is of the order of 3000.

6.3 Induced currents in the human body resulting from the proximity to surfaces at fixed potentials

A particularly important exposure scenario to study is when an operator in a power substation room raises his arm in order to touch a keyboard at a certain voltage V_0. Considering the worst case scenario of feet in contact with earth, the extended arm, which can be seen as a thin long aspect ratio highly conductive object, will facilitate the development of non-negligible currents throughout the body.

This section deals with a realistic parametric model of the grounded human body standing inside a power substation room, in order to estimate the current density along the body and how it varies as the person gets closer to the electrified panel, which represents the driver of the problem. In addition, the influence of the different shapes and conductivities of some selected organs on the numerical results obtained is estimated.

The physical model under study in these examples contemplates a grounded, isolated human being inside a power substation room, with an arm pointing to a keyboard at a fixed potential and the air in its near environment such as the case shown in Figure 6.4.

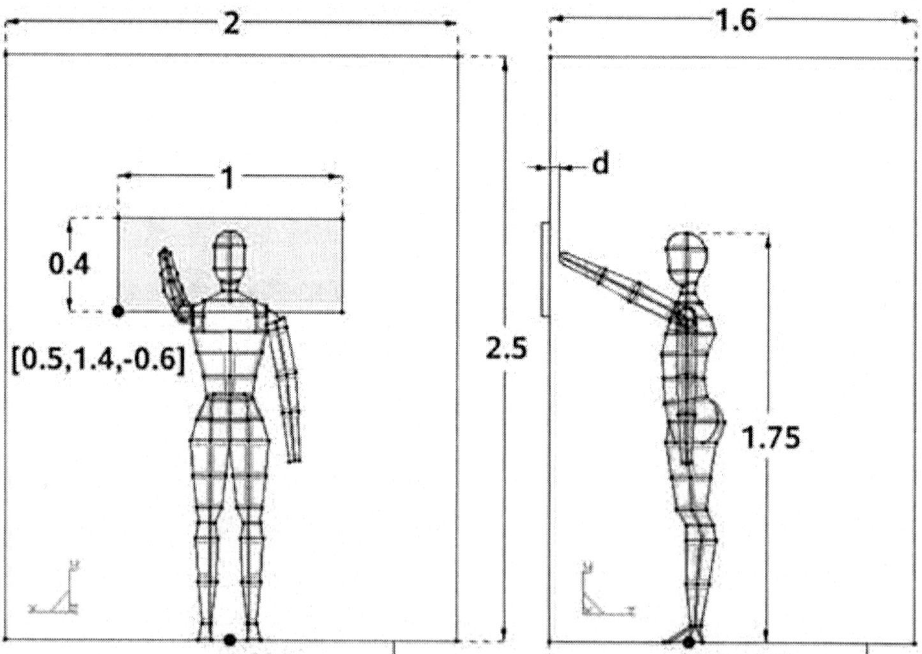

Figure 6.4: Main dimensions of the conceptual model representing a human body inside a substation room, extending his arm towards an electrified rectangular panel.

The room is modelled as a 2.5 m high, 1.6 m wide and 2 m long closed parallelepiped surrounding the human body as shown in Figure 6.4. The 1.75-m tall human being is facing a hypothetical control panel of 1 m wide and 0.4 m high at the level of the head. The lower right (right from the human body point of view) corner of the model is located at coordinates $(x, y, z) = (0.5, 1.4, -0.6)$ m, when taking into account the origin at the intersection between the vertical longitudinal axis of the human body and the ground floor, indicated as (0, 0, 0) in Figure 6.4.

Two different conditions will be evaluated on the basis of this model, namely A and B. The former considers a gap $d = 0.016$ m between the person's hand and the panel, while the latter is shifted 10 cm further away from the panel, i.e. $d = 0.116$ m. The gap is considered as a dielectric material (dry air). The boundary conditions applied are as follows. The panel has fixed potential $V_0 = 400$ V, while the floor is kept grounded and all other surfaces of the room are considered with Neumann adiabatic type conditions (i.e. $\nabla\varphi \cdot \hat{n} = 0$). Because of the linearity of the problem the results shown in this calculation can be scaled to any other value of applied voltage V_0.

In this example, two different conceptual models for the human body are considered, namely H and HO. H model is a homogeneous representation of the human body, while the HO model takes into account the presence of some relevant tissues like brain and heart. All organs are treated as conductors embedded in a saline fluid. Two sets of conductivity values have been considered for the organs, namely σ_L and σ_G. They are summarised in Table 6.2.

Table 6.2: Selected tissue conductivities in S/m at 60 Hz.

Tissue type	σ_L	σ_G
Embedding medium	0.50	0.35
Heart	0.11	0.10
Brain	0.12	0.06

Then, the induced current in the different conceptual models of the body at the two different scenarios and for both conductivity distributions is analysed for a total of eight datasets. Figure 6.5 shows one of the meshed models with 5038 flat linear triangular elements and 2506 nodes.

Figure 6.6 shows the absolute value of the current density $|\mathrm{j}| = \sqrt{j_x^2 + j_y^2 + j_z^2}$ along the vertical y-direction. The observation lines goes along the centroid of the crotch, torso, neck and head. The figure shows a comparison between the HO and H models at the smallest distance between hand and panel for both conductivity distributions. It can be observed that the consideration of rough approximations of the internal organs introduce slight modifications of the general behaviour predicted by the homogeneous model (H). The profile is mostly dominated by the external shape and exposure conditions and a second-order correction appears when keeping into account the organs. The presence of the heart introduces a fluctuation of nearly 0.2×10^{-2} mA/m^2 in the current density observed outside it. The consideration of the brain in the model introduces a similar deviation in the current density. In addition, the maximum peak of approximately 2.4×10^{-3} mA/m^2 is located near the waist, invariably where the cross section is slightly reduced. This behaviour suggests that the effect of a local depression on the sectional area normally exposed to the driving field is the most important factor that determines the profile of induced currents inside the body.

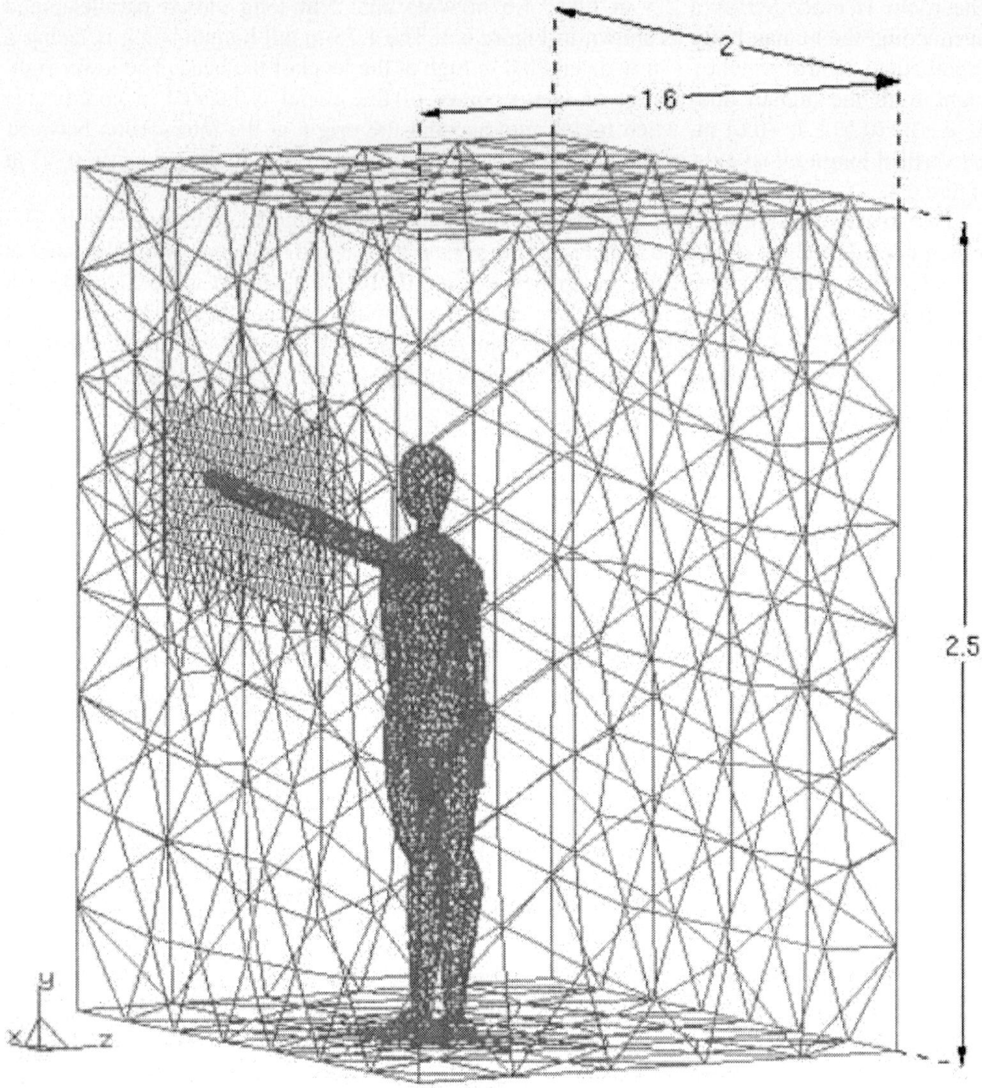

Figure 6.5: Boundary element mesh adopted for the model (5038 linear triangular elements).

Figure 6.7 shows the absolute value of the current density along the vertical *y* direction for the HO models at two different exposure scenarios for both conductivity distributions. As expected, current densities in scenario A are nearly 50% greater than that in B. Both conductivity distributions show nearly the same values of current density.

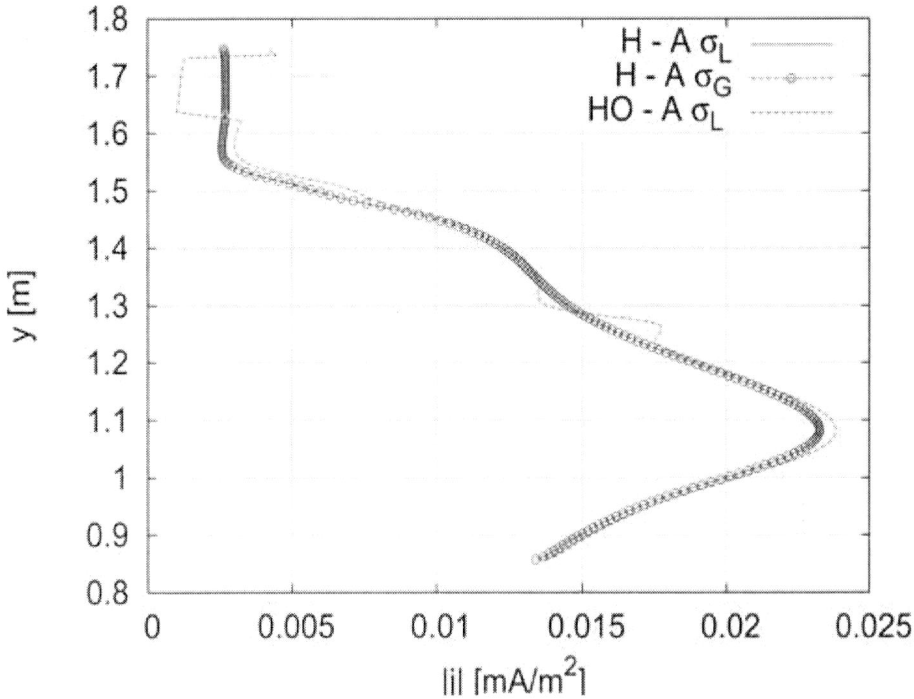

Figure 6.6: Absolute value of the current density along the torso for the H and HO models in the exposure scenario A for both conductivity distributions σ_L and σ_G.

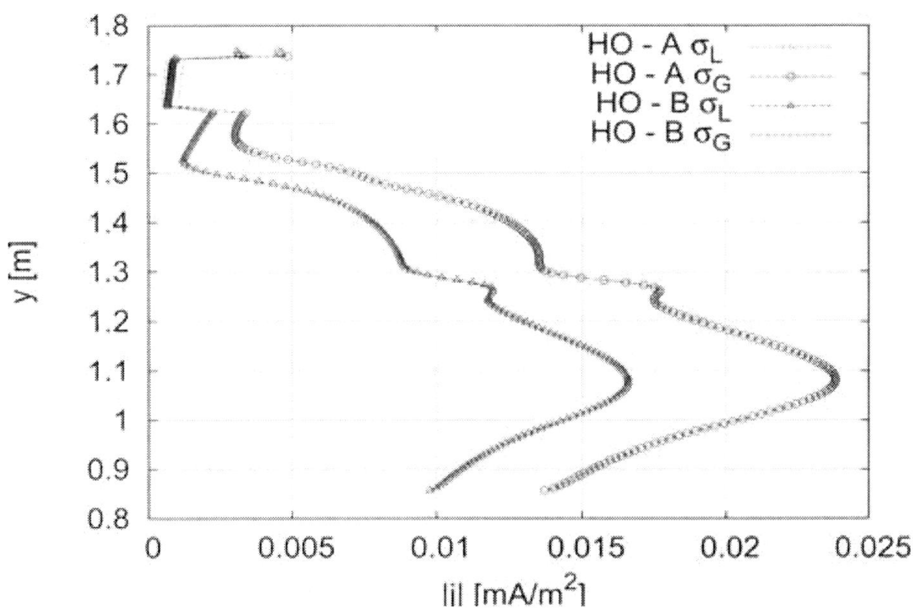

Figure 6.7: Absolute value of the current density along the torso for the HO model in the two different exposures scenarios A and B for both conductivity distributions σ_L and σ_G.

Figure 6.8 shows the absolute value of the current density inside the heart along the vertical *y*-direction for scenarios A and B, and both conductivity distributions. The current density in the heart decays roughly 1 μA/m^2 when shifted 10 cm away from the panel. The maximum absolute value of current density found in the heart is 3.2 μA/m^2 and 4.4 μA/m^2 for case scenario A and B, respectively. The values found are way below the recommended guidelines at ELF [2]. As expected, the current density induced under exposure scenario B is lower than that under scenario A. The values obtained for both conductivity distributions are similar for all the models considering organs and lower than the correspondent values for the homogeneous model H.

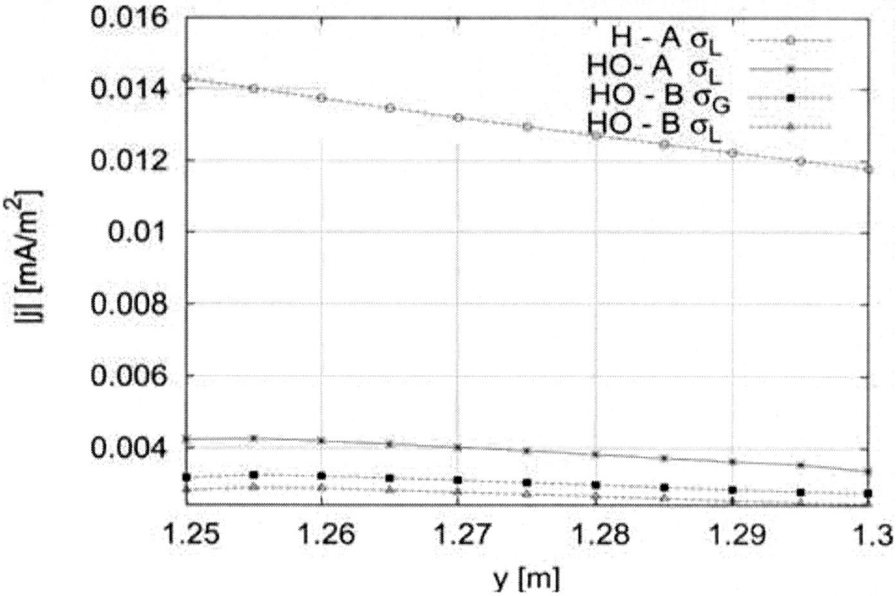

Figure 6.8: Absolute value of current density along the heart at the two exposure conditions and both conductivity distribution.

Finally, Figure 6.9 shows a 3D view of the current density distribution for the H model in scenario A. The arrows have constant length (i.e. they are not in scale with the values of current density, but show the main flow direction). The mostly exposed region of the body is the arm extended towards the panel, while the other one is basically unaffected.

6.4 Summary

The case study analysed in this chapter refers to the human body inside a power substation room, in different situations. Firstly, the exposure is analysed when the man is located in the interior of a substation room. Different exposure conditions have been considered for vertical, horizontal and oblique electric fields. The behaviour of the current density obtained in the case of the human body located in the vicinity of the transformer substation is consistent with the behaviour found in the case of transmission lines.

Secondly, the problem of a man with his arm extended towards a hypothetical electrified panel has been considered. The problem is driven by the voltage V_0 of this panel, which is assigned as a boundary condition.

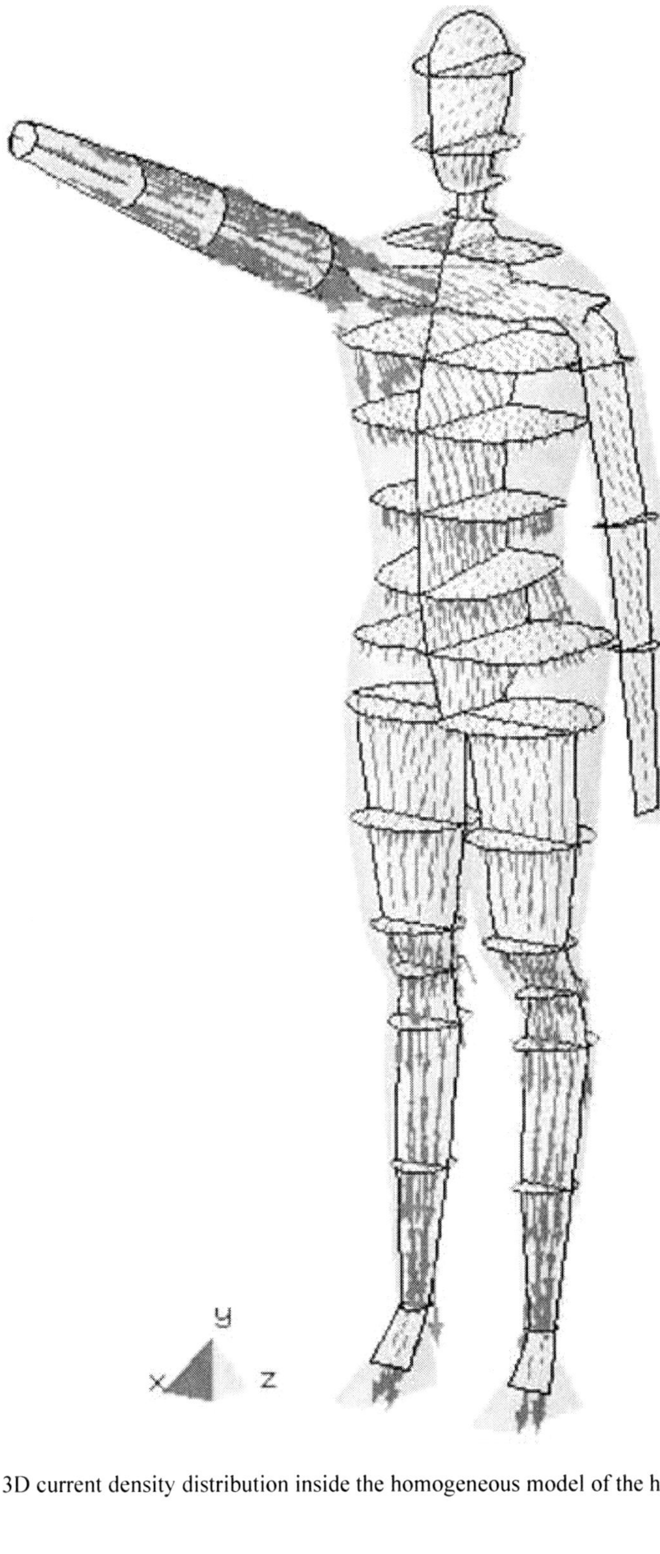

Figure 6.9: 3D current density distribution inside the homogeneous model of the human body.

The current density along the vertical axis of the body, when located at two different distances from the panel, has been accurately calculated for the case of grounded body and non-contacting conditions between hand and panel (i.e. the gap between hand and panel is air, in dry conditions).

The study reveals that the maximum peak of current occurs near the waist, around the region of reduced cross section. When the hand approximates the keyboard without touching it, considering a 1.6 cm gap of dry air in between, the maximum current density observed in the waist is approximately 2.4×10^{-2} mA/m^2, assuming a panel voltage $V_0 = 400$ V. Then, when shifted 10 cm apart, the maximum value decreases to nearly 1.6×10^{-2} mA/m^2.

The calculation has been repeated for a homogeneous human body with $\sigma \sim 0.5$ S/m and a heterogeneous one, which includes nearly ellipsoidal models of heart and brain with reduced conductivity ($\sigma \sim 0.11$ S/m). Two sets of conductivity values have been assigned to the different tissues. The overall result for the eight datasets calculated is nearly the same, except that the induced current inside those tissues is significantly modified. In all cases, the location and magnitude of the maximum peak of current density is mostly dominated by the external shape of the body, rather than by the distribution of internal non-homogeneous inclusions. Although the particular scenarios defined for the exposure studies described in this chapter cannot be compared with earlier publications, the values obtained for the current density and fields inside the body are in good agreement with the general results found in earlier publications under similar conditions [19, 25].

7

Pregnant woman

7.1 Introduction

Exposure levels in the foetus of a pregnant woman are difficult to estimate mainly because of the following three main factors. Firstly, the lack of data on electrical properties at low frequency for the foetus and the surrounding tissues; secondly, the impossibility of collecting in vivo measurements in a real case scenario and finally, because of the complicated changes in the geometrical and physical properties of body along the pregnancy period. Hence, a numerical modelling approach represents a powerful analysis tool, especially appealing when conducting sensitivity analysis on the electrical properties, which are scarce and scattered in the available literature. The aim of this chapter is to analyse the case of exposure of a pregnant woman to high-voltage overhead power lines by means of numerical techniques with BEM.

The analysis consists of measuring the induced currents and electric fields in the foetus in different scenarios of conductivities at different time stages of pregnancy and considering different presentations of the foetus inside the maternal matrix.

The differentiation in stages of pregnancies arises not only from the geometrical point of view, but also due to the variation of electrical properties of tissues during gestation. Since, as has been established in Chapter 3, amniotic fluid and foetus tissues are more conductive than adult tissues. These differences in conductivity values are suggesting that the modelling of the pregnant women including the amniotic fluid and the foetus tissues is necessary.

This chapter is divided into five sections and organised as follows. Section 7.2 describes the aspects considered for the implementation of the conceptual model based on the existing knowledge on the foetal development, the changes in the foetus and mother throughout gestation, anthropometric measures of the foetus as well as mother anatomy and foetus lie and presentation. Then, the geometry including the sub-domains (or compartments) of the model and the different scenarios of conductivities are established. Section 7.3 describes a BEM strategy, especially designed for minimising the number of degrees of freedom in this type of exposure models. Section 7.4 introduces the numerical implementation of the model, describes the conceptual model and summarises the different experiments that have been conducted. Section 7.5 presents the results obtained for the different case studies and their corresponding analysis.

7.2 Physical model

This section describes the assumptions considered in the development of the model of the pregnant woman and foetus and the different scenarios proposed for the calculation of induced electric fields, potentials and currents.

The development of the physical model involves two aspects, the geometrical model of the mother and foetus, and the *material* model, in which material properties are assigned to the geometrical model.

Therefore, it is necessary to have some insight in the changes that occur throughout gestation in order to correctly define the physical model. Different stages of pregnancy are modelled separately in order to consider the changes throughout gestation. These changes are related not only to the volume, mass and geometry of the maternal body and foetus, but also to the electrical properties of the participant tissues.

7.2.1 Foetal and embryo development

This section summarises background information [112] for foetal and embryo development, which was necessary for the definition of the conceptual models in this chapter.

Pregnancy is often divided into trimesters. The first 12 weeks correspond to the first trimester, 13–28 weeks to the second and 29 weeks to time of birth (generally the 40th week) to the third one. It is normally difficult to establish precisely the starting of the new life (fertilisation of the ovum), therefore the exact foetal age is practically impossible to determine. This is why the gestational age (measured in weeks) is more commonly used in obstetrics. Gestational age is estimated from the last menstrual period preceding fertilisation. However, in the literature, it may not always be clear which measurement criterion is applied. Fertilisation generally occurs approximately on day 14 of the menstrual cycle or in the second week of the gestational age.

In this way, the whole process of gestation is usually divided into several stages [112]: pre-gestation stage, which involves two weeks before fertilisation, pre-embryonic stage, after fertilisation and the stage when zygote experiences a process of cell divisions ending up in the formation of the blastocyst. During this period, the pre-embryo is transported from the ovary through the oviduct into the uterus for implantation into the uterine wall. Implantation is completed by the end of the second week. The period from the third to eighth week of the development is known as the embryonic period. The embryonic period is very important because this is the time when all internal and external structures develop in the embryo. In this period the different tissues and organs are developed. During this critical period, the exposure of an embryo to certain agents such as external EM fields may cause major congenital malformations.

The end of the embryonic stage occurs by the end of eighth week and then the foetal period begins. During the foetal period, the growth, development and maturation of the structures that have been already formed takes place. Henceforth, based on the different stages of the foetus evolution, the definition of the model reflects the four different stages of pregnancy spread along gestation. Finally, bearing these considerations in mind, the models adopted in this work correspond to the 8th, 13th, 26th and 38th gestational weeks.

7.2.2 Definition of sub-domains

As mentioned in Sections 3.6.4 and 3.6.5 of Chapter 3, the conductivity data for the foetus is scarce and scattered in the literature. For the maternal abdomen, the division into sub-domains is based on the different properties of the tissues. The amniotic fluid has the highest conductivity which varies depending on the period of gestation as discussed in Chapter 3. Tissues such as kidney, muscle bone cortical, bladder, spleen, cartilage and skin have all conductivity values very close to 0.1 S/m, ovary and cartilage have conductivity ~ 0.2 S/m.

Therefore, all these tissues can be grouped into one sub-domain, namely maternal tissue. Moreover, the uterus conductivity is 0.23 S/m, which is very similar to the conductivity of the maternal tissue. Hence, the uterus is incorporated into this sub-domain. In accordance with reference [49], the placenta is assumed to have the same conductivity as the blood. Thus, it is considered as part of the maternal-tissue sub-domain. A more accurate description of the placenta and how it participates in the electrical model will be addressed in future work. Consequently, the maternal abdomen is divided into three sub-domains namely 'maternal tissue', 'amniotic fluid', contained within the uterus and 'foetus'.

7.2.3 Geometrical definition

The geometrical definition for the foetus model was designed with the help of CT images of foetuses at different stages [113] and data on the anatomy of the mother and foetus were extracted from reference [46]. The most commonly anthropometric measurements for the size of the foetus are based on the crown-rump length (CRL) and the biparietal diameter (BPD). The CRL is defined as the greatest distance between the vertex of the skull and the ischial tuberosities, with the foetus in the natural curled position [46]. The BPD is the distance between the two biparietals and serves as a measure of the growth of the head. The BPD measurements show that growth is almost linear in the early weeks of pregnancy, but there is a progressive reduction in growth rate, especially during the final weeks. Another common foetal measurement is the abdominal diameter. Although not very common in obstetrics, the length of the leg available in the literature [112,113] for weeks 26 and 38 was also used to define the geometry. Additionally, reference values [46] of the surface area of the foetal body were included in the definition of the geometry of the foetus. Table 7.1 summarises data on the CRL, BPD and AD throughout the different stages considered.

Table 7.1: Anthropometric measurements for the foetus [cm].

Measurement	Week 8	Week 13	Week 26	Week 38
CRL	4.5	10	22	35
BPD	1.8	3	6	9
AD				3.5
Leg length			13	15
Surface area [cm^2]	27	250	850	230

During the foetal period, length and weight do not change in the same way. Foetal length change is greatest in the second trimester, while foetal weight change is greatest in the final weeks of development.

Furthermore, the foetus is free to move inside the maternal abdomen, principally until the 24th week. Since then, the movement is more constrained. In obstetrics, the foetal orientation and position are normally described in terms of the *foetal lie, presentation attitude* and *position*. The *foetal lie* describes the orientation of the longitudinal axe of the foetus in relation to the longitudinal axe of the mother. If the longitudinal axe of the foetus is parallel to the longitudinal axe of the mother, the foetus is in *longitudinal lie*, while if it is perpendicular or oblique, the foetus is in *transverse* or *oblique lie*, respectively. Longitudinal lie occurs in the 95% of the cases.

The foetal attitude describes the relative positions of different parts of the body of the foetus in relation with its own body. For example, in the most normal foetal attitude, referred as well as *the foetal position*, the head is tucked down to the chest, with arms and legs drawn in towards the centre of the chest.

The *presentation* of the foetus refers to his orientation in relation with the birth channel. The normal presentation is cephalic presentation, with the head oriented to the birth channel. When the foetus is in cephalic presentation and foetal position, then the presentation is referred to as *vertex presentation*. This presentation is the most common at delivery and occurs in the 96% of the births. Another presentation that occurs in the 3.5% of the births is the *breech presentation* when the buttocks are oriented towards the birth channel. The last and less frequent presentation (0.5%) is the *shoulder presentation* associated with transverse lie.

The modelling has considered these characteristics and included different presentations for the different gestational ages, which are summarised in Table 7.2. Figure 7.1 shows a view of the model developed for the 26 weeks foetus in the cephalic and breech presentations. The data for the maternal geometry and its variation along pregnancy is shown in Table 7.3 [46]. As can be seen, there is a change in the volume of amniotic fluid during gestation. During the first period of gestation, the amniotic fluid is generated by the maternal plasma, but as gestation advances, foetal urine contributes to the total volume of amniotic fluid. Moreover, there is a general increase of mass distributed over the maternal body [46].

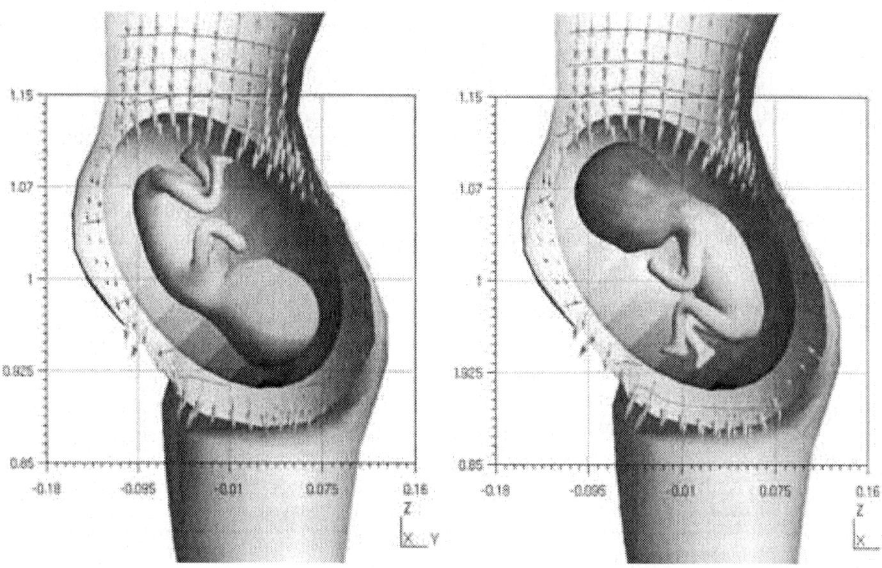

Figure 7.1: Geometrical model for the 26 weeks foetus in cephalic and breach presentations.

Table 7.2: Foetal presentations and lie considered in the model.

Position	Week 8	Week 13	Week 26	Week 38
Lie	Longitudinal for all the gestational ages			
Presentation	Cephalic	Cephalic	Cephalic	Vertex
Presentation	Breach	Breach	Breach	Complete

breach

Table 7.3: Anthropometric data for the pregnant woman.

Mass [g]	8 Week	13 Week	26 Week	38 Week
Foetus	4.7	160	990	3400
Placenta	–	50	430	650
Amniotic fluid	–	55	520	800
Uterus	50	200	450	970
Breasts	–	60	240	405
Blood	–	150	1000	1450
Extra cellular extra vascular fluid	0	10	50	1480
Unaccounted maternal stores	–	320	2900	3340
Total	55	1005	6580	12,500

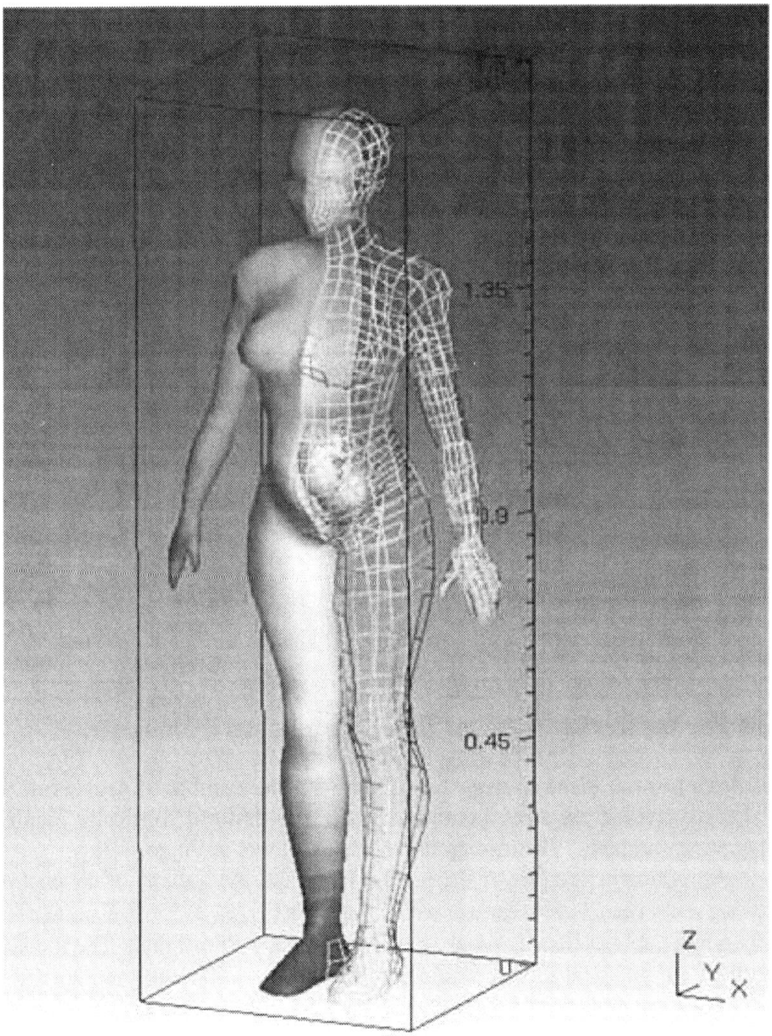

Figure 7.2: Geometrical model at 26 weeks of pregnancy in cephalic presentation.

Figure 7.2 shows a 3D view of the model at 26 weeks of pregnancy with the foetus in cephalic presentation. All the geometrical information was introduced by means of the open source 3D pre-processor Blender (www.blender.org). This software is oriented to CAD, animation and rendering in 3D space. To the best of the author's knowledge, it has never been used before for creating meshes for BEM. Moreover, the user interface and mesh generation is very appealing for BEM models of human tissues.

7.2.4 Modelling scenarios

This section describes the different scenarios that have been studied for the calculation of induced electric fields, potentials and currents in the model of the pregnant woman. The analysis is broken down into three parts in order to address the following three aspects:

Different scenarios of electrical conductivity: The tissue conductivity adopted for this analysis is chosen in accordance with the data and calculations performed in Chapter 3. In Chapter 3, foetal and maternal conductivities were estimated and the values used by Dimbylow [49] summarised. The three conductivities scenarios adopted in this work are summarised in Table 7.4, where σ_f refers to the foetus tissues conductivity, σ_{AF} to the amniotic fluid and σ_m to the maternal tissues conductivity.

Different time stages of pregnancy: Four different gestational ages are considered in this work corresponding to 8, 13, 26 and 38 weeks.

Different presentations of the foetus: Two different presentations have been considered for each gestational age. See Table 7.2.

Table 7.4: Conductivity scenarios.

Scenario	[S/m]	Week 8	Week 13	Week 26	Week 38
	σ_f	0.23	0.23	0.23	0.23
1	σ_{AF}	1.28	1.28	1.27	1.10
	σ_m	0.20	0.20	0.20	0.20
	σ_f	0.996	0.996	0.574	0.574
2	σ_{AF}	1.70	1.70	1.64	1.64
	σ_m	0.52	0.52	0.52	0.52
	σ_f	0.732	0.732	0.396	0.396
3	σ_{AF}	1.70	1.70	1.64	1.64
	σ_m	0.17	0.17	0.17	0.17

7.3 BEM for vertically incident field in open environments

This section describes the BEM strategy for minimising the number of degrees of freedom in the model of the grounded pregnant woman exposed to a uniform, vertically incident electric field in an open environment.[1] The conceptual model is shown in Figure 7.3(a).

The integration domain consists of the human body and the volume of air enclosed within the floor, ceiling and lateral walls represented by surfaces Γ_{FLOOR} at $z = 0$, Γ_{TOP} at $z = H$ and Γ_W at $\rho = a$, respectively, in a cylindrical system of coordinates with origin o. The top surface Γ_{TOP} is considered as an imaginary, flat, equipotential surface with constant voltage given by $\varphi(z = H) = V_0$, while the floor is at potential $\varphi(z = 0) = 0$.

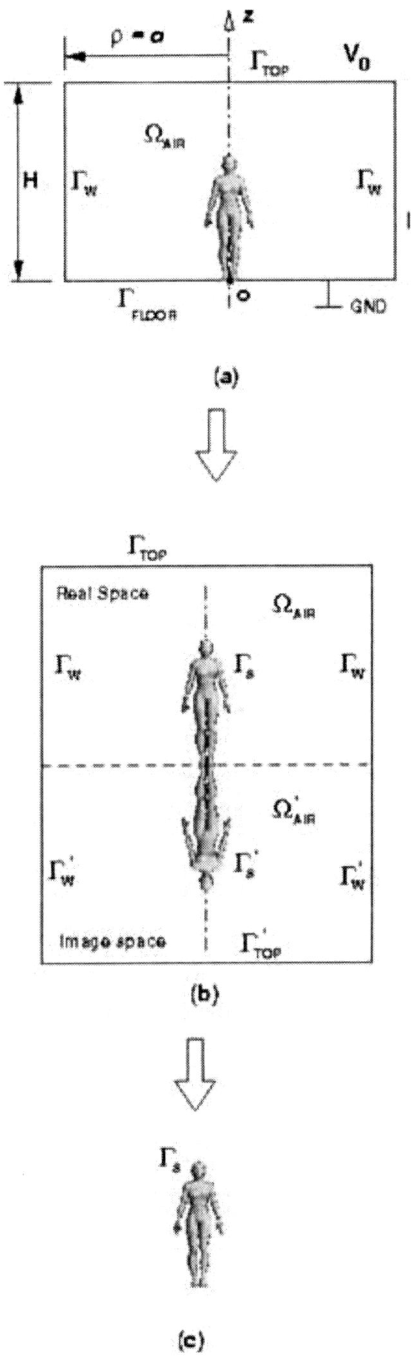

Figure 7.3: Simplification of the conceptual model. (a) Original conceptual model. (b) Floor discretisation is avoided by reflecting the problem. (c) Top and lateral wall discretisation is replaced with asymptotic analytical integrations.

In an open environment, the lateral walls Γ_w are assumed to be far from the body (i.e. $\rho = a \to \infty$) with potential given by the following equation:

$$\varphi\big|_{\text{wall}} = \frac{zV_0}{H} \tag{7.1}$$

hence, with normal electric field $E_n = 0$.

Because of the symmetry of the problem, it is possible to eliminate the discretisation of all the external boundaries by means of the following assumptions. The floor, considered as a perfectly conductive plane, can be eliminated by introducing an image space, as shown in Figure 7.3(b). The potentials and electric fields in the imaginary space are the same as those in the real space, but with opposite sign. Hence:

$$\varphi(x, y, z) = -\varphi(x, y, -z) \quad \text{and} \quad E_n(x, y, z) = E_n(x, y, -z). \tag{7.2}$$

In this way, the discretisation of the floor is no longer required and several hundreds of elements can be spared. In the next step, the discretisation of the lateral and top surfaces, as well as their corresponding images are also removed by analytical integration, thus saving more degrees of freedom. Finally, the discretisation for the external problem, i.e. involving the air and the human body, consists only of surface elements on the skin of the body. In this way, the level of discretisation is reduced and conveniently simplified leading to two main advantages: firstly, a reduction in the number of degrees of freedom of typically few thousand elements with respect to a standard model in which the body is inside a box and secondly, rather more technical, the model construction for changing shapes of human body becomes simpler, since the shape of the 'air', regarded as a sub-domain surrounding the body, does not need to be re-defined each time the skin changes its shape.

The rest of this section explains how the discretisation on lateral and top walls in both real and imaginary space can be eliminated by means of analytical integrations.

The integral equation for the potential φ in a point $\mathbf{x}_s \in \Omega_{air}$ located in the region of the air close to the body is given by:

$$c(\mathbf{x}_s)\varphi(\mathbf{x}_s) + \int_\Gamma \frac{\partial G(\mathbf{x}, \mathbf{x}_s)}{\partial n}\varphi(\mathbf{x})\mathrm{d}\Gamma - \int_\Gamma G(\mathbf{x}, \mathbf{x}_s)E_n(\mathbf{x})\mathrm{d}\Gamma = 0, \tag{7.3}$$

where G is the Green's function of Laplace equation, i.e.:

$$\nabla^2 G(\mathbf{x}, \mathbf{x}_s) + \delta(\mathbf{x}, \mathbf{x}_s) = 0, \tag{7.4}$$

$\Gamma = \partial(\Omega)$ is the boundary of the air surrounding the body, composed of the lateral walls Γ_w, the top surface Γ_{TOP} and the skin Γ_s including the real and imaginary space, i.e. $\Gamma = \Gamma_w \cup \Gamma_{TOP} \cup \Gamma_s \Gamma'_w \cup \Gamma'_{TOP} \cup \Gamma'_s$.

The aim is to take advantage of the symmetry and asymptotic behaviour of the solution of the problem in order to eliminate the mesh discretisation in Γ_W, Γ_{TOP} and Γ_{FLOOR}.

7.3.1 Analytical approach for lateral walls and top surface

The integration for the double and single layer potentials in Γ_W can be done in cylindrical coordinates as follows:

$$I_w^1 = \int_{\Gamma_w} \frac{\partial G(\mathbf{x}, \mathbf{x}_s)}{\partial n}\varphi(\mathbf{x})\mathrm{d}\Gamma = \int_{\theta=0}^{2\pi}\int_{z=0}^{H} \frac{-1}{4\pi\rho^2}\frac{zV_0}{H}\rho\,\mathrm{d}\theta\mathrm{d}z = -\frac{V_0 H}{4\rho}. \tag{7.5}$$

Therefore in the limit $\rho \rightarrow \infty$, the above integral tends to zero. In addition, the single layer potential integral becomes zero, since $E_n = 0$, i.e.

$$\int_{\Gamma_w} G E_n \mathrm{d}\Gamma = 0. \tag{7.6}$$

At the top surface the normal derivative of G becomes:

$$\frac{\partial G}{\partial n} = -\frac{\mathbf{r} \cdot \hat{n}}{4\pi r^3} = -\frac{H - z_s}{4\pi(\rho^2 + (H - z)^2)^{3/2}}, \tag{7.7}$$

where $r = ||\mathbf{x} - \mathbf{x}_s||$. The potential is fixed as follows:

$$\varphi = V_0, \tag{7.8}$$

and $\mathrm{d}\Gamma = \rho \mathrm{d}\rho \mathrm{d}\theta$. Therefore, the integral of the double layer potential is written as:

$$I_T^1 = \int_{\Gamma_{\mathrm{TOP}}} \frac{\partial G}{\partial n} \varphi \mathrm{d}\Gamma = \int_{\theta=0}^{2\pi} \int_{\rho=0}^{a} \frac{(z_s - H)V_0}{4\pi(\rho^2 + (H - z)^2)^{3/2}} \rho \mathrm{d}\rho \mathrm{d}\theta, \tag{7.9}$$

which results into the following equation:

$$I_T^1 = \frac{(z_s - H)V_0}{2} \left\{ \frac{-1}{\sqrt{a^2 + (H - z)^2}} + \frac{1}{|H - z|} \right\}, \tag{7.10}$$

then, in the limit $a \rightarrow \infty$, expression (7.10) becomes as follows:

$$\lim_{a \rightarrow \infty} \int_{\Gamma_{\mathrm{TOP}}} \frac{\partial G}{\partial n} \varphi \mathrm{d}\Gamma = -\frac{V_0}{2}. \tag{7.11}$$

By repeating these steps in the imaginary surface Γ'_{TOP}, the following result is obtained:

$$\lim_{a \rightarrow \infty} \int_{\Gamma'_{\mathrm{TOP}}} \frac{\partial G}{\partial n} \varphi \mathrm{d}\Gamma = \frac{V_0}{2}. \tag{7.12}$$

Finally, the two double layer potential integrals (7.11) and (7.12) cancel with each other, yielding the following equation:

$$\lim_{a \rightarrow \infty} \left\{ \int_{\Gamma_{\mathrm{TOP}}} \frac{\partial G}{\partial n} \varphi \mathrm{d}\Gamma + \int_{\Gamma'_{\mathrm{TOP}}} \frac{\partial G}{\partial n} \varphi \mathrm{d}\Gamma' \right\} = 0. \tag{7.13}$$

The integral of the single layer potential due to sources in the top surface of the real space is written as follows:

$$I_{\mathrm{TOP}} = \int G(\mathbf{x}, \mathbf{x}_s)\, E_n \mathrm{d}\Gamma, \tag{7.14}$$

where

$$G(\mathbf{x}, \mathbf{x}_s) = \frac{1}{4\pi r} = \frac{1}{4\pi\sqrt{\rho^2 + (H - z)^2}}, \tag{7.15}$$

$$\mathrm{d}\Gamma = \rho \mathrm{d}\theta \mathrm{d}\rho, \tag{7.16}$$

and

$$E_n = \nabla \varphi \cdot \hat{n} = \frac{V_0}{H}. \tag{7.17}$$

Therefore, I_{TOP} becomes as follows:

$$I_{\mathrm{TOP}} = \int_{\theta=0}^{2\pi} \int_{\rho=0}^{a} \frac{V_0 \rho}{4\pi H \sqrt{\rho^2 + (H-z)^2}} \mathrm{d}\rho \mathrm{d}\theta = \frac{V_0}{2H} \left[\sqrt{a^2 + (H-z)^2} - (H-z) \right]. \tag{7.18}$$

Analogously for the imaginary space, it results:

$$I'_{\mathrm{TOP}} = \int_{\theta=0}^{2\pi} \int_{\rho=0}^{a} \frac{-V_0 \rho}{4\pi H \sqrt{\rho^2 + (H+z)^2}} \mathrm{d}\rho \mathrm{d}\theta = -\frac{V_0}{2H} \left[\sqrt{a^2 + (H+z)^2} - (H+z) \right]. \tag{7.19}$$

Here, we are interested in the superposition of equations (7.18) and (7.19)

$$I_{\mathrm{TOP}} + I'_{\mathrm{TOP}} = \frac{V_0}{2H} \left\{ a \left[\sqrt{1 + \left(\frac{H-z}{a} \right)^2} - \sqrt{1 + \left(\frac{H+z}{a} \right)^2} \right] + 2z \right\}. \tag{7.20}$$

In the limit when $\alpha \rightarrow \infty$ the last expression becomes as follows:

$$\lim_{a \to \infty} \left[I_{\mathrm{TOP}} + I'_{\mathrm{TOP}} \right] = \frac{z V_0}{H}. \tag{7.21}$$

To summarise, when $\alpha \rightarrow \infty$, the integral equation (7.3) for the air sub-domain, can be replaced by the following equation:

$$c(\mathbf{x}_s)\varphi(\mathbf{x}_s) + \int_{\Gamma_S} \frac{\partial G(\mathbf{x}, \mathbf{x}_s)}{\partial n} \varphi(\mathbf{x}) \mathrm{d}\Gamma - \int_{\Gamma_S} G(\mathbf{x}, \mathbf{x}_s) E_n(\mathbf{x}) \mathrm{d}\Gamma = -\frac{z V_0}{H}, \tag{7.22}$$

which involves only two integrals in the skin surface of the body, one for the single layer potential and another for the double layer potential.

7.4 Numerical implementation

7.4.1 Conceptual model

The conceptual model consists of a homogeneous anatomical shape of pregnant woman (body) with the uterus and foetus immersed in it. The body is placed in an open environment, standing barefoot on a perfectly conductive infinite flat surface at $z = 0$, at ground level ($\varphi = 0$). This represents the worst case scenario for open environments in which currents throughout the body are expected to be maximum.

The pregnant woman is exposed to a reference field oriented in z direction, with asymptotic value $E_0 \hat{\mathbf{z}}$ when $z \rightarrow \infty$, as shown in Figure 7.3. These conditions are recreated by fixing an equipotential plane $\varphi = V_0$ at $z = H$, where H is sufficiently larger than the height of the woman and then scaling-up the results by a factor $\theta = H/V_0 \times E_0$, in order to translate the results into a particular magnitude of incident field E_0. In particular, in this chapter the results were obtained by adopting $V_0 = 1$ V and $H = 5$ m. Then, for example, in order to translate the results to the case of $E_0 = 10$ kV/m, a factor $\theta = 5 \times 10^7$ which multiplies j is adopted in order to obtain j in mA/m^2.

Table 7.5: Solving strategy. Connectivity between sub-domains and surfaces involved in the model of pregnant woman and boundary conditions applied to each surface. '×' symbol indicates an unknown of the problem.

Coupled model								
	Ω_{AIR}		Ω_{BODY}		Ω_{AF}		Ω_F	
	φ	E_n	φ	E_n	φ	E_n	φ	E_n
Γ_{TOP}	V_0	×	-	-	-	-	-	-
Γ_W	$\frac{zV_0}{H}$	0	-	-	-	-	-	-
Γ_{FLOOR}	0	×	-	-	-	-	-	-
Γ_{SA}	×	×	×	×	-	-	-	-
Γ_{SF}	-	-	0	×	-	-	-	-
Γ_{T1}	-	-	×	×	×	×	-	-
Γ_{T2}	-	-	-	-	×	×	×	×

=

Stage 1			
Ω_{AIR}		Ω_{BODY}	
φ	E_n	φ	E_n
V_0	$\frac{V_0}{H}$	-	-
$\frac{zV_0}{H}$	0	-	-
0	×	-	-
×	×	×	×
-	-	0	×
-	-	-	-
-	-	-	-

+

Stage 2					
Ω_{BODY}		Ω_{AF}		Ω_F	
φ	E_n	φ	E_n	φ	E_n
-	-	-	-	-	-
-	-	-	-	-	-
-	-	-	-	-	-
φ_s	E_{ns}	-	-	-	-
0	×	-	-	-	-
×	×	×	×	-	-
-	-	×	×	×	×

The BEM model consists of four sub-domains, Ω_{AIR}, Ω_{BODY}, Ω_{AF} and Ω_F, namely air, body, amniotic fluid and foetus, respectively. The air is bounded by Γ_{TOP}, Γ_W, Γ_{FLOOR} and Γ_S; while the body is bounded by Γ_s and Γ_{ti}, $i = 1, \ldots, N_t$, where Γ_{ti} represents the surface enclosing the different internal organs embedded in the homogeneous body and N_t is the number of organs. Part of Γ_S is in contact to the ground Γ_{SF}, while the rest is in contact to the air Γ_{SA}. Table 7.5 summarises the relationship between sub-domains, surfaces and boundary conditions in the model. The '×' symbol in the table indicates an unknown, while '–' symbol indicates that the corresponding surface is not related to the sub-domain.

The complete problem involves the air (considered as an external problem) and the body with its internal organs and the foetus. In order to reduce the computational burden as much as possible, the solution approach with BEM is split into two parts, corresponding to the internal and external problem. Hence, the BEM solving approach consists of two stages: 1 and 2.

Stage 1 solves the external problem, involving the air coupled to the homogeneous body (i.e. without internal tissues). The aim of Stage 1 is to find the electric field and potential in the skin, considering it as an interface separating air from body. Note that the inclusion of the body without internal tissues does not introduce significant errors in the results on the skin, as proved in Chapter 5, Section 5.7.2.

The values of potential and normal electric field obtained for the skin from the second stage are imposed as boundary conditions in order to solve the interior problem in the second stage. The interior problem consists of the body, amniotic fluid and foetus. The outcomes of the second stage are potentials and normal fluxes at the interfaces of the internal tissues, i.e. Γ_{T1} and Γ_{T2}. Finally, these fields are used in order to compute the solution for j, E and ϕ at internal observation points.

Finally, Table 7.6 shows a list of the models analysed in this chapter.

Table 7.6: Naming convention and summary of models.

Model	Week of pregnancy	Conductivity scenario	Presentation
B081D	8	1	Breech
B081U	8	1	Cephalic
B082D	8	2	Breech
B082U	8	2	Cephalic
B083D	8	3	Breech
B083U	8	3	Cephalic
B131D	13	1	Breech
B131U	13	1	Cephalic
B132D	13	2	Breech
B132U	13	2	Cephalic
B133D	13	3	Breech
B133U	13	3	Cephalic
B261D	26	1	Breech
B261U	26	1	Cephalic
B262D	26	2	Breech
B262U	26	2	Cephalic
B263D	26	3	Breech
B263U	26	3	Cephalic
B381D	38	1	Breech
B381U	38	1	Cephalic
B382D	38	2	Breech
B382U	38	2	Cephalic
B383D	38	3	Breech
B383U	38	3	Cephalic

7.5 Results and discussion

Figure 7.4 shows a lateral view of the sliced model of the pregnant woman. The direction of the electric field in the maternal tissues is shown by black arrows. The iso-lines represent the electric potential field.

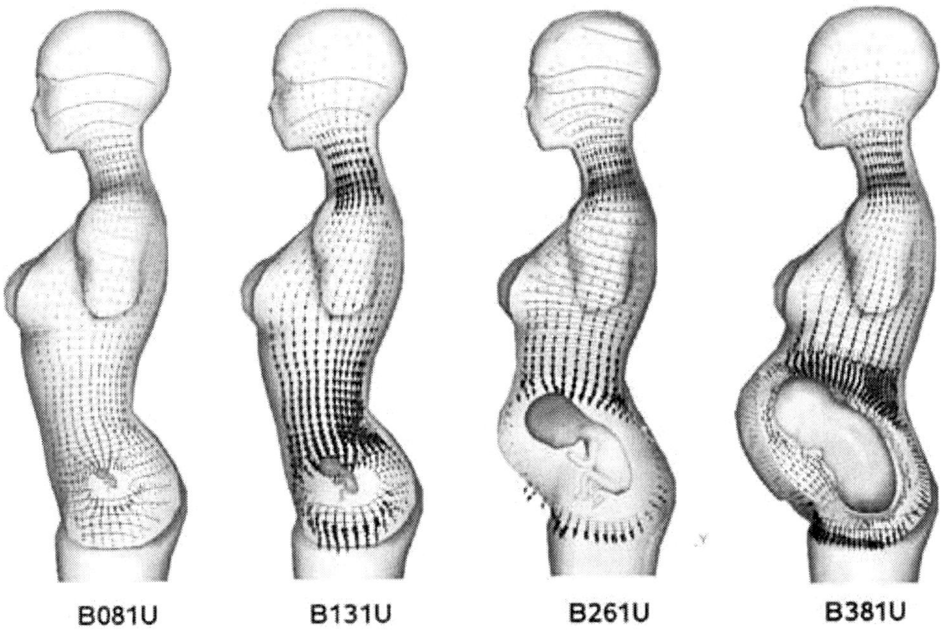

Figure 7.4: Lateral view.

Figure 7.5 shows a 3D view of the sliced model of the pregnant woman including some of the results obtained for the potential and electric field. The model is partially sliced with clipping planes in order to visualise the interior results. There are seven colour bars on the left hand side of the figure which show the correspondence between the colour map and the numerical scale in each case. All results correspond to the case of exposure to 1/5 V/m. 'U_body0' corresponds to the potential observed inside the model in the sagittal plane, excluding the limbs. 'U_foetus' refers to the potential measured in the skin of the foetus. The values range from 1.41 to 1.34 μV. 'U_skin' corresponds to the potential measured in the maternal skin, i.e. the interface between air and body. The maximum value ~2 μV is obtained near the head, while the minimum ($\sim O(10^{-3}$ μV)) is in the nearest part of the skin contacting the soil (feet). 'E_body' and 'E_body0' correspond to the vector field plot representing the electric field in the internal part of the maternal body. The former, ranging from 0.74 to ~0.02 μV/m, refers to the coronal sectioning plane including arms and legs, while the latter, ranging from ~2 to ~0.02 μV/m refers to the sagittal planes excluding limbs. Finally, 'U_uterus' and 'U_body' indicate the potential in the uterus and body surfaces, respectively. It can be observed how the uterus tends to concentrate the field lines. This is because of its higher conductivity with respect to the maternal tissue.

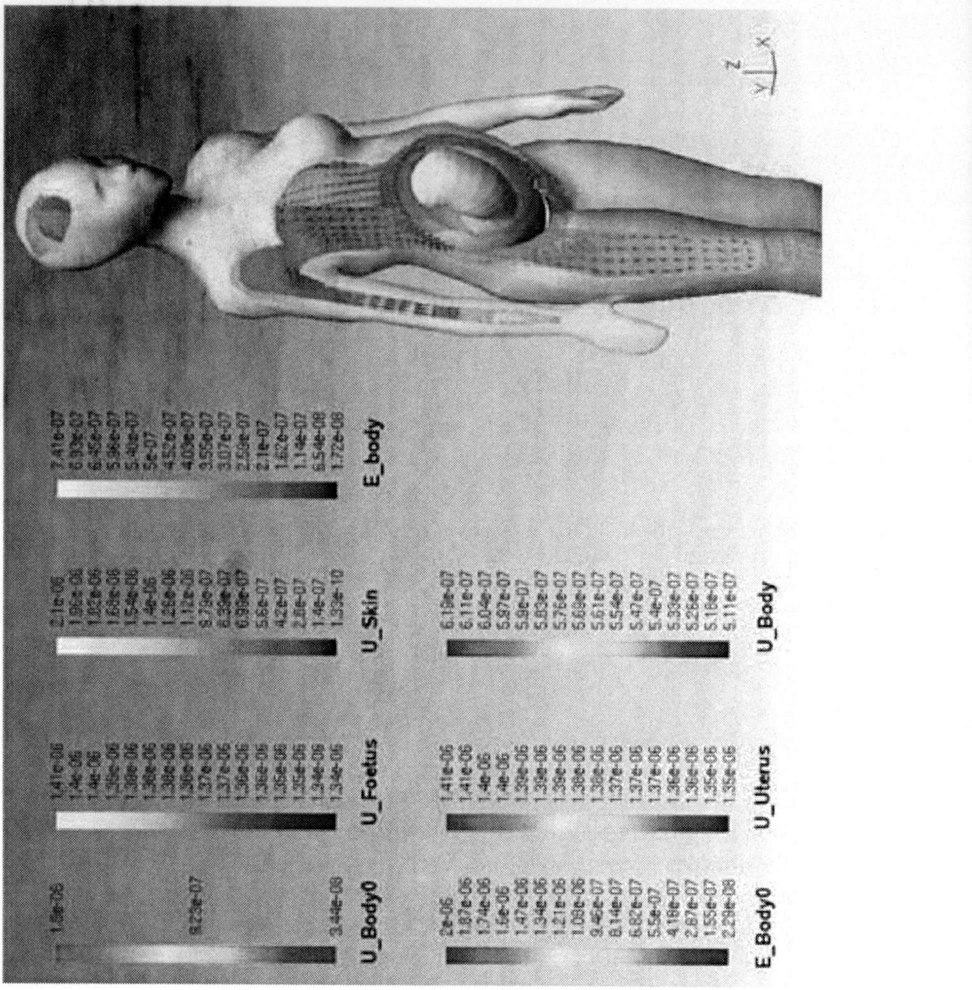

Figure 7.5: Electric field in V/m per 0.25 V/m.

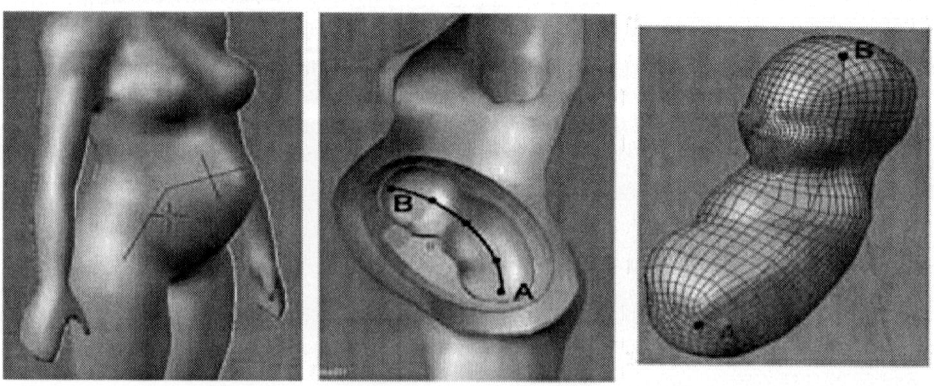

Figure 7.6: Observation line along the spine of the foetus.

7.5.1 Current density along the foetus

Figure 7.6 shows the observation line that goes along the spine of the foetus, where the current density has been measured. Figure 7.7 shows |**J**| in function of z along the observation line AB inside the foetus. The incident field has been scaled to 10 kV/m and the currents are expressed in mA/m^2. The figure illustrates the numerical findings at different weeks of pregnancy in the three different conductivity scenarios. Each plot compares the same results for two different presentations of the foetus: cephalic and breech.

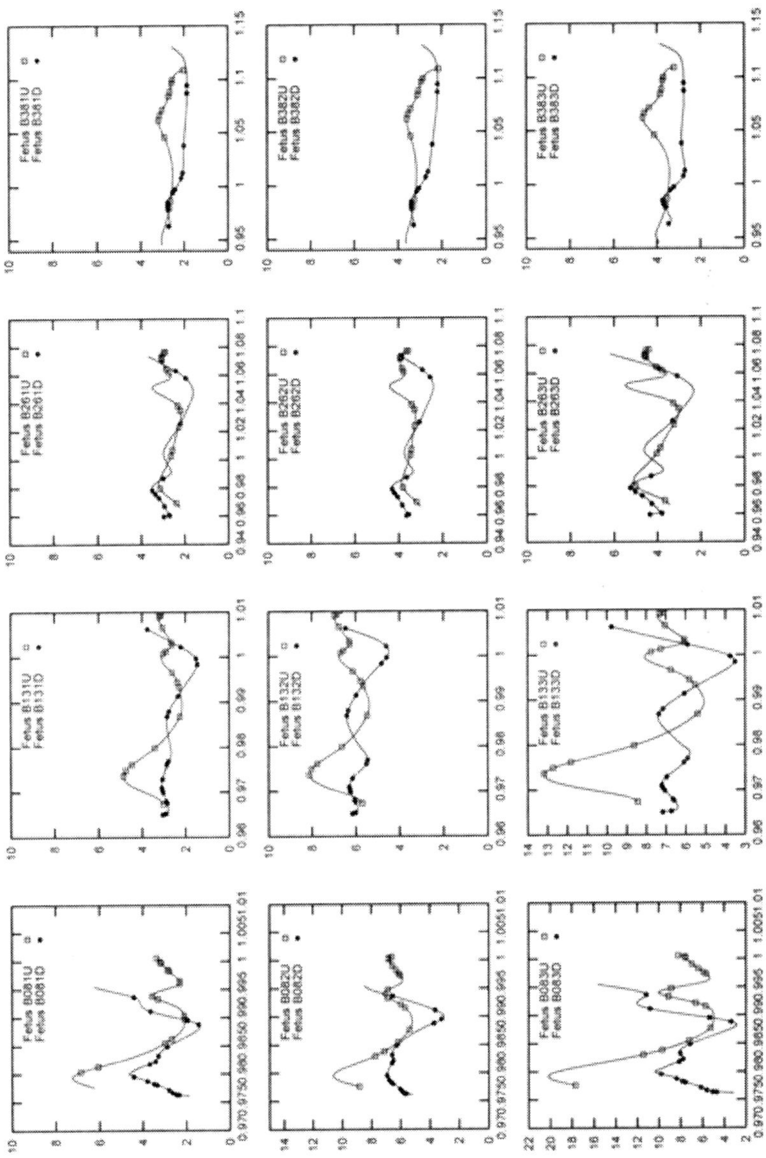

Figure 7.7: Current density along the spine of the foetus. Scenarios 1, 2 and 3. Ages: 8, 13, 16 and 38 weeks.

Each row in Figure 7.7 corresponds to a particular conductivity scenario (i.e. first row corresponds to scenario 1, and so on), while each column corresponds to a particular gestational age (i.e. first column represents 8th week, 2nd to 13th week, 3rd to 26th and 4th to 38th week).

7.5.1.1 Current density variation throughout gestation

Along a row in Figure 7.7, the maximum values of current density are obtained at the eighth gestational week and then it decreases progressively as the foetus develops. This behaviour is observed in the three scenarios. The decrease of current density flowing through the foetus with age can be explained as a consequence of the two following factors. First, the foetus conductivity as well as the amniotic fluid conductivity decrease with age. Second, as the foetus grows, he tends to adopt a *vertex presentation* (extremities drawn in towards the centre of the chest and head tucked down to the chest), hence his external surface is smoother and the cross-sectional area becomes more regular.

7.5.1.2 Differences in current density between conductivity scenarios

Along a column, it is possible to compare the current density for a particular age at different conductivity scenarios. Figure 7.8 illustrates the relation between foetal and maternal tissue conductivity for each scenario and gestational age organised in the same order that in Figure 7.7.

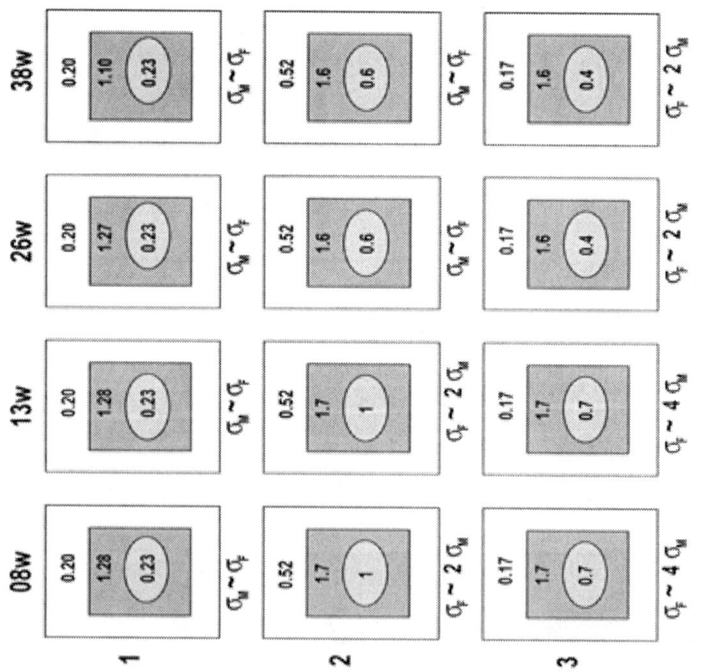

Figure 7.8: Scenarios illustration showing the relation between maternal and foetus conductivities.

The current flows preferentially through pathways of high conductivity. The amniotic fluid conductivity is more or less high and constant in different scenarios and gestational ages. Therefore, the relation between maternal and foetal tissues conductivities will contribute to determine the pathways of current.

From Figure 7.7, for all gestational ages, it is observed that the current density in the foetus in the case of scenario 3 is bigger than in scenario 2 and in scenario 2 is bigger than scenario 1. However, the high contrast in current densities observed between scenarios in weeks 8 and 13 is attenuated in weeks 26 and 38. This behaviour can be explained by considering the ratios between foetal and maternal conductivities shown in Figure 7.8.

In the case of scenario 1, foetal conductivity is similar to maternal tissues conductivity, while for scenarios 2 and 3 foetal conductivity is bigger.

Therefore, the current density in scenario 3 is expected to be bigger than in scenario 2 and the latter bigger than in scenario 1.

However, in scenario 2 (and 3), weeks 8 and 13, the foetus conductivity is approximately 2 (and 4) times bigger than the maternal tissue conductivity, respectively. On the other hand, for weeks 26 and 38, the foetus conductivity is approximately similar (and 2 times bigger) than the maternal conductivity. Therefore, the contrast in current densities between scenarios is attenuated in week 26 and 38.

7.5.1.3 Current density variation with the presentation of the foetus

The comparison of current densities induced in the foetus, between the two different presentations considered (breech and cephalic), shows that for all scenarios and gestational ages the breech presentation gives higher current densities along the body of the foetus. This effect is less pronounced in the last stage of pregnancy (38 week).

This can be explained by considering that the part of the body with bigger cross-sectional area (i.e. the head) is exposed to a higher field when the foetus is in breech presentation, thus giving rise to higher currents flowing along the body.

As the foetus grows, he tends to adopt the *foetal position* attitude. This makes his cross-sectional area to become more homogeneous. Hence, the difference in current density between the two presentations becomes less pronounced.

7.5.2 Mean and extreme values of current density in the foetus

Figures 7.9–7.11 show the mean, maximum and minimum values of current density computed in the foetus at different weeks of pregnancy. The results compile the maximum and minimum values of current density ($j = \sigma_f|\nabla\varphi|$) calculated along the spine of the foetus, including the two different presentations: cephalic and breech.

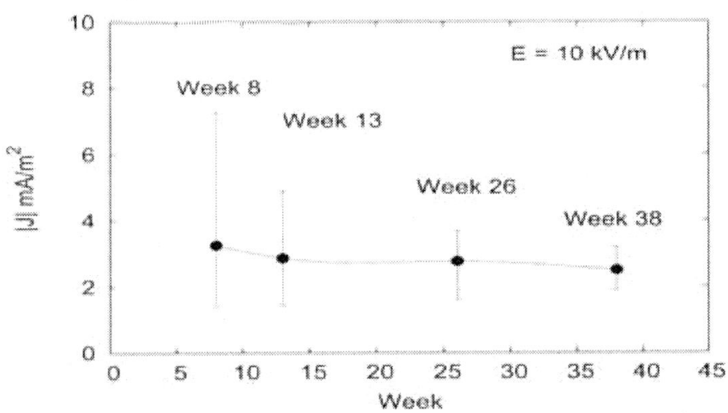

Figure 7.9: Mean current density calculated in the foetus at weeks: 8, 13, 26 and 38 of pregnancy. Scenario 1.

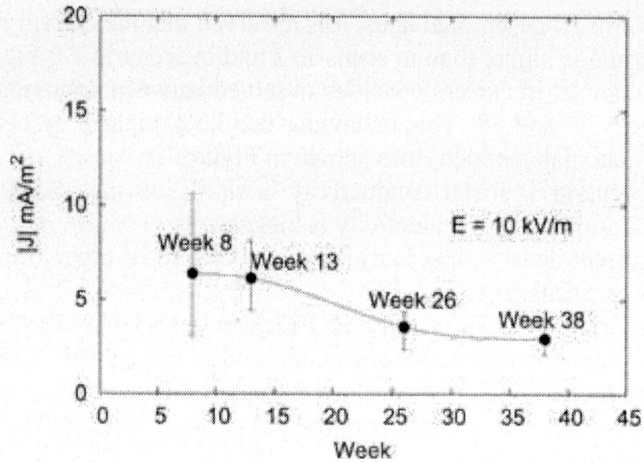

Figure 7.10: Mean current density calculated in the foetus at weeks: 8, 13, 26 and 38 of pregnancy. Scenario 2.

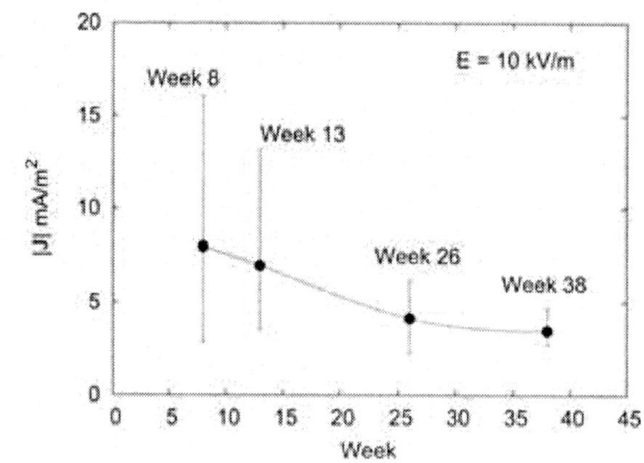

Figure 7.11: Mean current density calculated in the foetus at weeks: 8, 13, 26 and 38 of pregnancy. Scenario 3.

It can be observed that the variation of current density inside the foetus decreases with age. This is due to the increasing uniformity of the foetus model, where the geometry is smoother and less fluctuations are expected in the results.

7.5.3 Dosimetry analysis

According to the results shown in Figures 7.9–7.11, the maximum value of current density in the foetus occurs during the 8th week. The maximum current density obtained in the foetus for an incident external field of 10 kV/m is 7.4 mA/m^2. On the other hand, the restriction recommended for public exposure by ICNRP [2] is 2 mA/m^2. Then, this restriction translates into a maximum external field $E_1 = 2.7$ kV/m. Table 7.7 generalises this analogy for the three scenarios studied, by showing the equivalent electric fields restrictions. The first three columns indicate the current densities obtained in the foetus at eighth week for an incident electric field of 10 kV/m in the three different scenarios. The last three columns indicate the external electric field that should be applied in order to measure a current density of 2 mA/m^2 in the foetus. The first row corresponds to the maximum values while the second to the average ones. According to these results, the mean values give a restriction for the electric field of approximately 3 kV/m based on the current circulating in the foetus, while the current restriction suggests approximately 50 kV/m, if it is based only on the maternal brain. Finally, Figure 7.12 shows the current density for the woman in the brain.

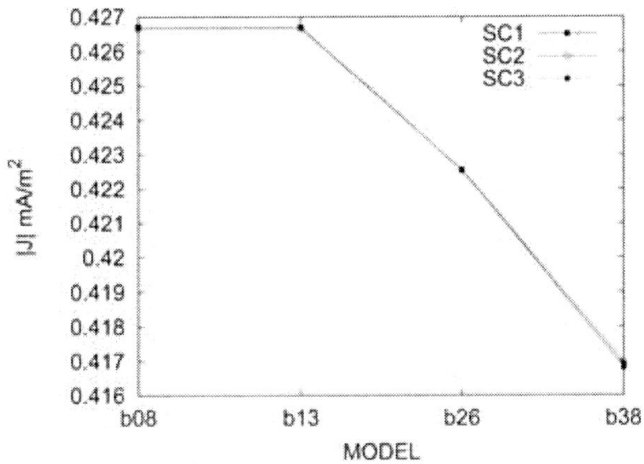

Figure 7.12: Current density along the maternal brain in all scenarios.

Table 7.7: Dosimetry analysis.

	Current density in foetus at 10 kV/m [mA/m^2]			External field restriction for $j = 2$ mA/m^2 in foetus [kV/m]		
	Scenario			Scenario		
	1	2	3	1	2	3
Maximum	7.4	10.7	17	2.70	1.87	1.18
Typical	3.2	5.8	7.5	6.25	3.45	2.67

7.6 Summary

This chapter has introduced a 3D anatomical multi-domain model of a pregnant woman and foetus at four different stages of pregnancy. The definition of the different physical and geometrical properties of the most relevant for each sub-domain was established according to the medical information available in the literature. The case of exposure to overhead power transmission lines was solved with the developed BEM method. The results obtained for the different stages of pregnancy are in good agreement with the results published in the existing literature [49]. A test matrix of different scenarios involving three sets of conductivity, two foetus postures and four pregnancy stages was proposed and solved. The results allowed to obtain mean values as well as maximum and minimum deviations of induced currents and electric fields in the foetus. The contrast of conductivity between foetus, amniotic fluid and maternal tissue is a key factor for the magnitude of induced currents in the foetus.

Note

1 This strategy can be equally applied to any other highly conductive object exposed to a vertically incident electric field.

8

Conclusions

8.1 Concluding remarks

The behaviour of electric fields and induced currents in the human body exposed to different scenarios of ELF high-voltage–low-intensity EM fields has been analysed by means of improved BEM. The general modelling approach in this work is based on 3D anatomical models, i.e. the kind of models which can be built by means of geometry modellers such as parametric CAD (computer aided design) software. This approach is somehow in the middle between oversimplified semi-analytical models and highly detailed anatomy-based models, such as those obtained from MRI images with sub-millimetre resolution.

The advantage of this intermediate approach resides in its capability of gaining comprehensive understanding while retaining as much as possible the details relevant to the physics of the problem. In addition, the relatively low-computational burden facilitates the systematic analysis of a variety of case scenarios. This is an appealing feature for conducting sensitivity analysis.

In this work, the coupling between air and biological tissues was carried out by considering natural matching conditions, i.e. by imposing the continuity of potentials and charge conservation across interfaces. Thus, avoiding the need to introduce artificial approximations such as the usual approach of imposing zero potential in the grounded human body model. Hence, the calculation allowed to compute small voltage differences occurring in the skin of the body.

With respect to the computational modelling aspects, a novel BEM strategy, namely S-BEM has been introduced. The S-BEM is based on mixing continuous and discontinuous nodes. This enables simpler assembly schemes (especially in multi-domain 3D models) and allows higher accuracy than the standard BEM with discontinuous elements.

In addition, a new analytical integration scheme for the single- and double-layer potentials has helped to speed up the calculations in the pre-processing and assembly schemes with respect to the classical BEM, leading at the same time to more accurate results. In particular, the integration method remains highly accurate even when the internal observation point approaches to the field boundary element of the domain (near singular case).

The developed methodology has been applied to three different case studies: (i) overhead power transmission lines, (ii) power substation rooms and (iii) pregnant woman.

The results obtained in all cases allowed to identify situations of high and low exposure in the different parts of the body and to compare with existing exposure guidelines. In the case of overhead power lines, a sensibility analysis considering the orientation of arms towards the incident field, as well as the effect of the inclusion of internal organs in the model on the total current density have been conducted. Results were compared to the classical simplified cylindrical models developed in the past.

It has been demonstrated that although oversimplified models, such as the ellipsoidal or cylindrical ones, are reasonably good for providing the correct understanding of the problem and the orders of magnitude involved, they underestimate the peaks of currents which appear whenever the cross-section exposed to the field is reduced. For example, they fail to represent correctly the peaks of current density which appear in neck and ankles in the case of vertical incidence of electric fields on a grounded human body.

Results can be compared with the basic restrictions established in reference [2]. As a reference, the ICNIRP establishes a maximum value of 10 mA/m^2, in case of exposure to ELF fields of frequency between 4 Hz and 1 kHz for head and trunk in the working population and 2 mA/m^2 for general public. The results found in this work, excluding the neck, are below the limit for working population; however proximity to the radiation source may easily increase this value.

8.1.1 Pregnant woman

Research in numerical modelling addressing the problem of exposure of pregnant woman to ELF EM fields is very limited at the moment. In addition, there is not enough information on the electrical properties of the foetus and surrounding tissues. This is why the combination of numerical modelling and sensitivity analysis with respect to the geometry and electrical properties has been adopted as a case for study in this work.

The results obtained for the different stages of pregnancy are in good agreement with the results published in the existing literature [49]. Hence, it was proved that the BEM becomes not only adequate but also convenient and efficient for solving anatomical models of pregnant woman exposed to ELF EM fields. The degree of detail achievable with this method is compatible, to a reasonable extent, with the current knowledge on electrical properties of the tissues involved.

In general, the results obtained allow to conclude that the contrast between foetus, amniotic fluid and maternal tissue conductivities plays a significant role in determining the magnitude of induced currents in the foetus. In addition, the detailed geometry of the foetus and its relative posture in the uterus are both important factors which should be kept into consideration when computing induced fields and currents in the foetus.

The results obtained for the pregnant woman reveal that the foetus is exposed to higher values of current density than the current in the brain of mother. In addition, the dosimetry analysis based on these results allow us to suggest that the current restriction in the electric field should be decreased to 3 kV/m in order to obtain a current density in the foetus below 2 mA/m^2 during the eighth week of gestational age.

Bibliography

[1] N. Siauve, R. Scoretti, N. Burais, L. Nicolas, and A. Nicolas. Electromagnetic fields and human body: a new challenge for the electromagnetic field computation. *Compel: Int. J. Comput. Math. Electr. Electron. Eng.*, 22(3): 457–69, 2003.

[2] ICNIRP. Guidelines for limiting exposure to time-varying electric, magnetic, and electromagnetic fields (up to 300 GHz). *Health Physics.*, 74(4): 494–522, 1998.

[3] A. Albohm, E. Cardis, A. Green, M. Linet, D. Savitz, and A. Swerdlow. Review of the epidemiologic literature on EMF and health. *Environ. Health Perspect.*, S6: S109, 2001.

[4] M.P. Maslanyj, T.J. Mee, D.C. Renew, J. Simpson, P. Ansell, S.G. Allen, and E. Roman. Investigation of the sources of residential power frequency magnetic field exposure in the UK childhood cancer study. *J. Radiolo. Prot.*, 27: 41–58, 2007.

[5] G. Draper, T. Vincent, M.E. Kroll, and J. Swanson. Childhood cancer in relation to distance for high voltage power lines in England and Wales: a case-control study. *Br. Med. J.*, 330(10), 2005.

[6] P. Fews, D. Henshaw, P. Keitch, J. Close, and R. Wilding. Increased exposure to pollutant aerosols under high voltage power lines. *Int. J. Radiat. Biol.*, 75: 1505–21, 1999.

[7] P. Fews, D. Henshaw, and P. Keitch. Corona ions from powerlines and increased exposure to pollutant aerosols. *Int. J. Radiat. Biol.*, 75: 1523–31, 1999.

[8] M.J. Crumpton and A.R. Collins. Are environmental electromagnetic fields genotoxic? *DNA Repair*, 3(10): 1385–7, 2004.

[9] S. Ivancsits, E. Diem, H.W. Rdiger A. Pilger, and O. Jahn. Induction of DNA strand breaks by intermittent exposure to extremely-low-frequency electromagnetic fields in human diploid fibroblasts. *JCMOSS*, 519(1–2): 1–13, 2002.

[10] M. Landgrebe, S. Hauser, B. Langguth, U. Frick, G. Hajak, and P. Eichhammer. Altered cortical excitability in subjectively electrosensitive patients: results of a pilot study. *J. Psychosom. Res.*, 62(3): 283–8, 2007.

[11] M. Roslia et al. Symptoms of ill health ascribed to electromagnetic field exposure a questionnaire survey. *Int. J. Hyg. Environ. Health*, 207(2): 141–50, 2004.

[12] E. Lyskov, M. Sandstrm, and K.H. Mild. Neurophysiological study of patients with perceived electrical hypersensitivity. *Int. J. Psychophysiol.*, 42(3): 233–41, 2001.

[13] EU. Risk evaluation of potential environmental hazards from low frequency electromagnetic field exposure using sensitive in vitro methods. Technical report, Contract: QLK4-CT-1999-01574, 2004. A project funded by the European Union under the programme Quality of Life and Management of Living Resources Key Action 4 “Environment and Health”.

[14] D. Graham-Rowe. ‘Conclusive’ study of cellphones fuels controversy. http://www.newscientist.com/article.ns?id=dn6819, December 2004. NewScientist.com news service.

[15] R. Plonsey and D.B. Heppner. Considerations of quasistationarity in electrophysiological systems. *Bull. Math. Biophy.*, 29: 657–64, 1967.

[16] M. Potter, M. Okoniewski, and M.A. Stuchly. Low frequency finite difference time domain (FDTD) for modeling of induced fields in humans close to line sources. *J. Comput. Phys.*, 162(1): 82–103, 2000.

[17] T.W. Dawson, K. Caputa, and M.A. Stuchly. High-resolution organ dosimetry for human exposure to low-frequency electric fields. *IEEE Trans. Power Del.*, 13(2): 366–73, 1998.

[18] T.W. Dawson, J. de Moerloose, and M.A. Stuchly. Comparison of magnetically induced ELF fields in humans computed by FDTD and scalar potential FD codes. *ACES J.*, 11: 63–71, 1996.

[19] A. Chiba, K. Isaka, Y. Yokoi, M. Nagata, M. Kitagav, and T. Matsuo. Application of finite element method to analysis of induced current densities inside human model exposed to 60 Hz electric field. *IEEE Trans. Power Apparatus Sys.*, 103(7): 1895–901, 1984.

[20] A. Peratta, C. Gonzalez, and D. Poljak. Current density induced in the human body due to power distributions lines using the boundary element method. *J. Comm. Soft.Syst.*, 3(1): 11–16, 2007.

[21] C. Gonzalez, A. Peratta, and D. Poljak. Current density induced in the human due to power distributions lines using the boundary element method. In *13th Int. Conf. on Software, Telecomm and Comp. Networks IEEE*, Split CROATIA, pp. 63–7, 2005.

[22] C. Gonzalez, A. Peratta, and D. Poljak. Boundary element modeling of the realistic human body exposed to extremely low frequency (ELF) electric fields: computational and geometrical aspects. *IEEE Trans. Electromagn. Compat.*, 49(1): 153–62, 2007.

[23] D. Poljak, C.Y. Tham, O. Gandhi, and A. Sarolic. Human equivalent antenna model for transient electromagnetic exposure. *IEEE Trans. EMC*, 45(1), 2003.

[24] R.W.P. King. A review of analytically determined electric fields and currents induced in the human body when exposed to 50–60 Hz electromagnetics fields. *IEEE Trans. Antennas Propag.*, 52(5): 1186–92, 2004.

[25] O.P. Gandhi and J.Y. Chen. Numerical dosimetry at power line frequencies using anatomically based models. *Bioelectromagnetics Suppl.*, 1: 43–60, 1992.

[26] C.M. Furse and O.P. Gandhi. Calculation of electric fields and currents induced in millimeter-resolution human model at 60 Hz using the FDTD method. *Bioelectromagnetics*, 19: 293–9, 1998.

[27] T.W. Dawson, J. de Moerloose, and M.A. Stuchly. Hybrid finite-difference method for high resolution modelling of low-frequency electric induction in humans. *J. Comp. Phys.*, 136: 640–53, 1997.

[28] T.W. Dawson and M.A. Stuchly. High-resolution organ dosimetry for human exposure to low-frequency magnetic fields. *IEEE Trans. Magnetics*, 34(3): 708–18, 1998.

[29] P.J. Dimbylow. Induced current densities from low frequency magnetic fields in a 2 mm resolution, anatomically realistic model of the body. *Phys. Med. Biol.*, 43: 221–30, 1998.

[30] M.A. Stuchly, O.P. Gandhi. Interlaboratory comparison of numerical dosimetry for human exposure to 60 Hz electric and magnetic fields. *Bioelectromagnetics*, 21: 167–74, 2000

[31] O.P. Gandhi, G. Kang, and G. Lazzi. Currents induced in anatomic models of the human for uniform and nonuniform power frequency magnetic fields. *Bioelectromagnetics*, 22: 112–21, 2001.

[32] O.P. Gandhi and G. Kang. Calculation of induced current densities for humans by magnetic fields from electronic surveillance devices. *Phys. Med. Biol.*, 46: 2757–71, 2001.

[33] T.W. Dawson, K. Caputa, and M.A. Stuchly. Numerical evaluation of 60 Hz magnetic induction in the human body in complex occupational environments. *Phys. Med. Biol.*, 44: 1025–40, 1999.

[34] P.J. Dimbylow. Current densities in a 2 mm resolution anatomically realistic model of the body induced by low frequency electric fields. *Phys. Med. Biol.*, 45: 1013–22, 200.

[35] A. Hirata, K. Kaputa K., T.W. Dawson, and M. Stuchly. Dosimetry in models of child and adults for low-frequency electric field. *IEEE Trans. Biomed. Eng.*, 48: 1007–12, 2001.

[36] P.J. Dimbylow. Development of the female voxel phantom, NAOMI, and its application to calculations of induced current densities and electric fields from applied low frequency magnetic and electric fields. *Phys. Med. Biol.*, 50: 1047–70, 2005.

[37] C.A. Brebbia, J.C. Telles, and L.C. Wrobel. *Boundary Elements Techniques*. Springer-Verlag, Berlin, Heidelberg New York and Tokio, 1984.

[38] Y. Shiau and A.R. Valentino. ELF electric field coupling to dielectric spheroidal models of biological objects. *IEEE Trans. Biomed. Eng.*, 28: 429–37, 1981.

[39] Kuane and McCreary. Numerical calculation and measurement of 60 Hz current densities induced in an upright grounded cylinder. *Bioelectromagnetics*, 6: 209–20, 1985.

[40] R. Spiegel. Numerical determination of induced currents in humans and baboons exposed to 60 Hz electric fields. *IEEE Trans. Electromagnetic Compatibility*, 24: 382–90, 1981.

[41] K.M. Chen, H.R. Chuang, and C.J. Lin. Quantification of interaction between ELF-LF electric fields and humans bodies. *IEEE Trans. Biomed. Eng.*, 24: 382–90, 1986.

[42] P. Dimbylow. Finite difference calculations of current densities in a homogeneous model of a man exposed to ELF electric fields. *Bioelectromagnetics*, 8: 355–75, 1987.

[43] J.G. Zubal, C.R. Harrel, E.O. Smith, Z. Rattner, G.R. Gindi, and P.H. Hoffer. Computerized three dimensional segmented human anatomy. *Med. Phys. Biol.*, 21: 299–302, 1994.

[44] T.W. Dawson, K. Caputa, and M.A. Stuchly. Influence of human model resolution of computed currents induced in organs by 60 Hz magnetic fields. *Bioelectromagnetics*, 18: 478–90, 1997.

[45] U.A. Fill, M. Zankl, N. Peoutssi-Hens, M. Siebert, and D. Regulla. Adult female voxel models of different stature and photon conversion coefficient for radiation protection. *Phys. Med. Biol.*, 86: 253–72, 2004.

[46] ICRP 2002. Basic anatomical and physiological data for use in radiological protection: reference values. *ISNN 0146-6453*, 89, 2002.

[47] T. Nagaoka, S. Watanabe, M. Taki, and Y. Yamanaka. Development of realistic high-resolution whole body voxel models of Japanese adult male and female of average height and weight, and application of models to radio-frequency electromagnetic field dosimetry. *Phys. Med. Biol.*, 49: 1–15, 2004.

[48] J. Chen. Mathematical models of the embryo and fetus for use in radiological protection. *Health Phys.*, 86: 285–95, 2004.

[49] P.J. Dimbylow. Development of pregnant female, hybrid voxel mathematical models and their application to the dosimetry of applied magnetic and electric fields at 50 Hz. *Phys. Med. Biol.*, 51: 2383–94, 2006.

[50] C.H. Durney, H. Massoudi, and Iskander. *Radiofrequency Radiation Dosimetry Handbook*. Brooks Air Force Base- USAFSAM-TR, pp. 85–73, 1986.

[51] J.D. Jackson. *Classical Electrodynamics*. J. Willey & Sons, New York, 1975.

[52] D. Poljak, A. Peratta, and C. Brebbia. The boundary element electromagnetic-thermal analysis of human exposure to base station antennas radiation. *Eng. Anal. Bound. Elem.*, 3(5), 2004.

[53] H.H. Pennes. Analysis of tissue and arterial blood temperature in resting forearm. *J. App. Physiol.*, 1: 93–102, 1948.

[54] A. Hiratta, M. Morita, and T. Shiozawa. Temperature increase in human head due to a dipole antenna at microwave frequencies. *IEEE Trans. Electromag. Compat.*, 35(1): 109–116, 2003.

[55] O.P. Gandhi, Xiang L.I., and G. Kang. Temperature rise for the human head for cellular telephones and for peak SARs prescribed in safety guidelines. *IEEE Trans. Microwave Theory Tech.*, 49(9): 1607–13, 2001.

[56] P. Fews, D. Henshaw, P. Keitch, J. Close, and R. Wilding. Increased exposure to pollutant aerosols under high voltage power lines. *Int. J. Radiat. Biol.*, 75: 1505–21, 1999.

[57] P. Schawn. Linear and nonlinear electrode polarisation and biological materials. *Ann. Biomed. Eng.*, 20: 269–88, 1992.

[58] P. Schawn. Electrical properties of tissues and cell suspensions. *Adv. Phys. Med. Biol.*, 5: 147–209, 1957.

[59] P. Schwan and K.R. Foster. RF-field interactions with biological systems: electrical properties and biophysical mechanisms. *Proc. IEEE*, 68: 104–13, 1980.

[60] K.R. Foster and H.P. Schwan. Dielectric properties of tissues and biological materials: a critical review, critical reviews in biomedical engineering. *Rev. Biomed. Eng.*, 17: 25–104, 1989.

[61] K.R. Foster. Thermal and nonthermal mechanisms of interaction of radio-frequency energy with biological systems. *IEEE Trans. Plasma Sci.*, 28(1): 15–23, 2000.

[62] M.J. Peters, J. Stinstra, and M. Hendriks. Estimation of the electrical conductivity of human tissue. *Electromagnetics.*, 21: 545–57, 2001.

[63] D. Miklavcic, N. Pavselj, and F. Hart. *Electric Properties of Tissues*. Wiley Encyclopedia of Biom. Eng., John Wiley and Sons, New York, 2006.

[64] M. Pavlin, T. Slivnik, and D. Miklavcic. Effective conductivity of cell suspensions. *IEEE Trans. Biomed. Eng.*, 49(1): 77–80, 2002.

[65] M.A. Stuchly and S.S. Stuchly. Dielectric properties of biological substances – tabulated. *J. Microwave Power*, 15(1): 19–26, 1980.

[66] C. Gabriel, S. Gabriel, and E. Corthout. The dielectric properties of biological tissues: I. Literature survey. *Phys. Med. Biol.*, 41: 2231–49, 1996.

[67] S. Gabriel, R.W. Lau, and C. Gabriel. The dielectric properties of biological tissues: III. Parametric models for the frequency spectrum of tissues. *Phys. Med. Biol.*, 41: 2271–93, 1996.

[68] C. Gabriel. Dielectric properties of biological tissue: variation with age. *Biolelectromagnetics*, 26(7): 1–18, 2005.

[69] H.F. Cook. The dielectric behaviour of some types of human tissues at microwave frequencies. *Brit. J. App. Phys.*, 2: 295–300, 1951.

[70] H.F. Cook. A comparison of the dielectric behaviour of pure water and human blood at microwave frequencies. *Brit. J. App. Phys.*, 3: 249–55, 1952.

[71] S. Gabriel, R.W. Lau, and C. Gabriel. The dielectric properties of biological tissues: II. Measurements in the frequency range 10 Hz to 20 GHz. *Phys. Med. Biol.*, 41: 2251–69, 1996.

[72] R. Chiu and M.A. Stuchly. Electric fields in bone marrow substructures at power line frequencies. *IEEE Trans. Biom. Eng.*, 52(6): 1103–9, 2005.

[73] B.R. Epstein and K.R. Foster. Anisotropy in dielectric properties of skeletal muscle. *Med. Biol. Eng. Comput.*, 21: 51–5, 1983.

[74] D. Haemmerich, O.R. Ozkan, J. Tsai, S.T. Staelin, S. Tungjitkusolmun, and D.M. Mahvi, and J.G. Webster. Changes in electrical resistivity of swine liver after occlusion and postmortem. *Med Biol. Eng. Comput.*, 40: 29–33, 2002.

[75] K.S. Cole. *Membranes, Ions and Impulses.* University of California Press, Berkeley, 1992.

[76] T.J.C. Faes, H.A. van der Meij, J.C. De Munck, and R.M. Heethaar. The electric resistivity of human tissues (100 Hz–10 MHz): a meta-analysis of review studies. *Physiol. Meas.*, 20: R1–R10, 1999.

[77] J.C. Maxwell. *A Treatise of Electricity and Magnetism.* Vol. 1, arts 311–314, New York, Dover, 1891.

[78] F. De Luca, C. Cametti, G. Zimatore, B. Maraviglia, and A. Pachi'. Use of low-frequency electrical impedance measurements to determine phospholipid content in amniotic fluid. *Phys. Med. Biol.*, 41(6): 1863–9, 1996.

[79] Y. Lu, H. Cui, J. Yu, and S. Mashimo. Dielectric properties of human fetal organ tissues at radio frequencies. *Bioelectromagnetics*, 17: 425–6, 1996.

[80] H. Kawai, K. Ito, M. Takahashi, K. Saito, T. Ueda, M. Saito, H. Ito, H. Osada, Y. Koyanagi, and K. Ogawa. Simple modeling of an abdomen of pregnant women and its application to SAR estimation. *IEEE Trans. Comm.*, 17: 3401–10, 2006.

[81] A. Peyman, A.A. Rezazadeh, and C. Gabriel. Changes in the dielectric properties of rat tissue as a function of age at microwave frequencies. *Phys. Med. Biol.*, 46(6): 1617–29, 2001.

[82] A.D. Bocking and R. Harding. *Fetal Growth and Development.* Cambridge University Press, 2001.

[83] C.A. Brebbia and J. Dominguez. *Boundary Elements, An Introductory Course.* 2nd edition. Computational Mechanics Publications, McGraw-Hill, New York Colorado San Francisco Springs Mexico Montreal Oklahoma City San Juan Toronto, 1992.

[84] J.J. do Rego Silva. *Acoustic and Elastic Wave Scattering Using Boundary Elements.* Vol. 18. Computational Mechanics Publications, Southampton UK and Boston USA, 1994.

[85] Sladek and Sladek, eds. *Singular Integrals in Boundary Element Methods.* Wit Press, 1996.

[86] V. Sladek, J. Sladek, and M. Tanaka. Evaluation of $1/r$ integrals in BEM formulations for 3D problems using coordinate multitransformations. *Eng. Anal. Bound Elem.*, 20: 229–44, 1997.

[87] V. Sladek and J. Sladek. Singular integrals and boundary elements. *Comput. Methods Appl. Mech. Eng.*, 157: 251–66, 1998.

[88] M. Guiggiani and A. Gigante. A general algorithm for multidimensional Cauchy principal value integrals in the boundary element method. *J. Appl. Mech.*, 57: 906–15, December 1990.

[89] M. Bonnet and M. Guiggiani b. Direct evaluation of double singular integrals and new free terms in 2D (symmetric) Galerkin BEM. *Comput. Methods Appl. Mech. Eng.*, 192: 25652596, 2003.

[90] A. Salvadori. Analytical integrations of hypersingular kernel in 3D BEM problems. *Comput. Methods Appl. Mech. Eng.*, 190: 3957–75, 2001.

[91] X. Gao. Evaluation of regular and singular domain integrals with boundary-only discretisation: theory and fortran code. *J. Comput. Appl. Math.*, 175: 265–90, 2005.

[92] X. Gao. Numerical evaluation of two-dimensional singular boundary integrals: theory and fortran code. *J. Comput. Appl. Math.*, 188: 44–64, 2006.

[93] D.E. Medina and J.A. Liggett. Exact integrals for three-dimensional boundary element potential problems. *Commun. Appl. Numer. Methods*, 5: 555–61, 1989.

[94] E. Allgower, K. Georg, and K. Kalik. Computation of weakly and nearly singular integrals over triangles in r^3. *preprint:1991*, pp. 1–10, 1991.

[95] R. Srivastava and D. Contractor. Efficient evaluation of integrals in three-dimensional boundary element method using linear shape functions over plane triangular elements. *Appl. Math. Modell.*, 16: 282–90, June 1992.

[96] K. Hayami. A numerical quadrature for nearly singular boundary element integrals. *Eng. Anal. Boundary Elem.*, 13: 143–54, 1994.

[97] H. Ma and N. Kamiya. Distance transformation for the numerical evaluation of near singular boundary integrals with various kernels in boundary element method. *Eng. Anal. Boundary Elem.*, 26: 329–39, 2002.

[98] Z. Niu, W.L. Wendland, X. Wang, and H. Zhou. A semi-analytical algorithm for the evaluation of the nearly singular integrals in three-dimensional boundary element methods. *Comput. Methods Appl. Mech. Eng.*, 194: 1057–74, 2005.

[99] A. Taigbenu. Simulation of coupled nonlinear electromagnetic heating with the green element method. In B. Sunden and C. Brebbia, eds. *Advanced Computational Methods in Heat Transfer IX*. Vol. 53 of *Engineering Sciences*. Wessex Institute of Technolgy, WIT Press, 2006.

[100] A. Taigbenu. *TheGreen Element Method*. Kluwer, Boston, USA, 1999.

[101] M. Ramsak, L. Skerget, M. Hribersek, and Z. Zunic. A multidomain boundary element method for unsteady laminar flow using stream functionvorticity equations. *Eng. Anal. Boundary Elem.*, 29(1): 1–14, 2005.

[102] A. Peratta and V. Popov. Hybrid BEM for the early stage of unsteady transport process. *Int. J. Numer. Methods Eng.*, 2006. In press.

[103] E. Anderson, Z. Bai, C. Bischof, S. Blackford, J. Demmel, J. Dongarra, J. Du Croz, A. Greenbaum, S. Hammarling, A. McKenney, and D. Sorensen. *LAPACK Users' Guide*. 3rd edition. Society for Industrial and Applied Mathematics, Philadelphia, PA, 1999.

[104] M.H. Repacholi, D. Noble, and A.F. McKinlay. Effects of static magnetic fields relevant to human health. pages –, Chilton, UK, 2004.

[105] R.W.P. King. Currents and electric fields induced in the human body when the arms are raised. *J. Appl. Phys.*, 81(11): 7116–28, 1997.

[106] R.W.P. King and S.S. Sandler. Electric fields and currents induced in organs of the human body when exposed to ELF and VLF electromagnetic fields. *Radio Sci.*, 31: 1153–67, 1996.

[107] Y. Saad. SPARSKIT: A basic tool kit for sparse matrix computations. Technical Report RIACS-90-20, Research Institute for Advanced Computer Science, NASA Ames Research Center, Moffett Field, CA, 1990.

[108] Youssef Saad. *Iterative Methods for Sparse Linear Systems*. Manchester University Press, Massachusetts, 1992.

[109] D. Poljak, A. Peratta, and C.A. Brebbia. A 3D BEM modelling of human exposure to ELF electric fields. In *Boundary Elements XXVII, Incorporating Electrical Engineering and Electromagnetics*. Orlando, EEUU, pp. 441–51, 2005.

[110] O.P. Gandhi. Some numerical methods for dosimetry: extremely low frequencies to microwave frequencies. *Radio Sci.*, 30(1): 161–77, 1995.

[111] N. Kovac, D. Poljak, S. Kraljevic, and B. Jajac. Computational of maximal electric field value generated by a power substation. In *BEM-MRM 28*, Skyatos, Greece, 2006.

[112] MJT FitzGerald MJT and M. FitGerald. *Human Embryology*. W. B. Saunders Company, London, 1994.

[113] UNSW Embriology – Dr. Mark Hill. Website.

[114] V. Amoruso, G. Calo, F. Lattarulo, D. Poljak, A. Peratta, and C. Gonzalez. A comparative study on the induce current density in humans exposed to ELF electric fields. *J. Comm. Soft. Syst.*, 3(1): 17–25, 2007.

[115] C. Gonzalez, A. Peratta, and D. Poljak. Human body exposure to fixed potential surfaces in power substations. In *Trans. on Biomed. and Health.* Vol. 12. Wessex Institute of Technology, Southampton UK, , pp. 24–252, 2007.

[116] C. Gonzalez, A. Peratta, and D. Poljak. Induced currents in the human body resulting from the proximity to surfaces at fixed potenials. In *15th Int. Conf. on Software, Telecomm and Comp. Networks. IEEE*, Split CROATIA, 2007.

[117] A. Peratta, C. Gonzalez, and D. Poljak. Geometrical aspects of 3D human body exposed to extremely low frequency electromagnetic fields. In *14th Int. Conf. on Software, Telecomm and Comp. Networks. IEEE*, Split CROATIA, 2006.

[118] D. Poljak, N. Kovac, C. Gonzalez, A. Peratta, and S. Kraljevic. Assessment of human exposure to power substation electric field. In *14th Int. Conf. on Software, Telecomm and Comp. Networks IEEE*, Split CROATIA, 2006.

[119] D. Poljak, C. Gonzalez, and A. Peratta. Assessment of human exposure to extremely low frequency electric fields using different body models and the boundary element analysis. In *18th Int. Conf. on Applied Electromagnetics and Communications. IEEE.* Vol. 14, Barcelona SPAIN, 2006.

[120] D. Poljak, A. Peratta, and C. Gonzalez. Human body response to extremely low frequency electric fields. In *EMC National Session*, Paris France, 2005.

[121] GID resources. Website.

[122] Blender. Website.

[123] CIMNE, International Center for Numerical Methods in Engineering, Barcelona, Spain. *GID, The personal pre/postprocessor Manual.*

[124] R. Lohner and P. Parikh. Generation of three-dimensional unstructured grids by the advancing front method. *Int. J. Numer. Methods Fluids*, 8: 1135–49, 1988.

[125] Ramon Ribó Rodríguez. *Desarrollo de un sistema integrado para tratamiento de geometría de malla y datos para el análisis por el método de los elementos finitos*. PhD thesis, Universitat Politécnica de Catalunya, 2000.

[126] C. Geuzaine and J-F. Remacle. Gmsh v 2.0. Reference Manual. http://www.geuz.org.

Appendices

Appendix A: Auxiliary primitives

$$\int \frac{\rho}{\sqrt{\rho^2 + c^2}} d\rho = \sqrt{\rho^2 + c^2} + C \tag{A1}$$

$$\int \frac{e\sqrt{e^2 + t^2 + c^2}}{e^2 + t^2} dt = c \arctan\left(\frac{ct}{e\Lambda_1}\right) + e\log(t + \Lambda_1) + C \tag{A2}$$

$$\int \frac{\rho^2}{\sqrt{(\rho^2 + c^2)^{3/2}}} d\rho = \log\left(\rho + \sqrt{c^2 + \rho^2}\right) - \frac{\rho}{\sqrt{c^2 + \rho^2}} + C \tag{A3}$$

$$\int \frac{\rho}{(\rho^2 + c^2)^{3/2}} d\rho = -\frac{1}{\sqrt{c^2 + \rho^2}} + C \tag{A4}$$

$$\int \frac{e}{(e^2 + t^2)\sqrt{c^2 + e^2 + t^2}} dt = \frac{1}{\mathrm{c}} \arctan\left(\frac{c\,t}{e\Lambda_1}\right) + C \tag{A5}$$

Note: C Є R is an arbitrary constant, and $\left[\Lambda_1 = \sqrt{c^2 + e^2 + t^2}\right]$.

Appendix B: Implementation notes

The pre-processing of the models, including mesh generation and geometry modelling, has been carried out by adapting existing pre-processing software: GID [121] and Blender [122]. The former is a general pre- and post-processing finite element oriented tool, while the latter is a general purpose scene simulation and rendering software from the open source community. In the GID-based approach, the geometrical information is introduced in a hierarchical way. First, a 3D wireframe is built out of a network of splines in order to define the main structure of the model. Second, closed loops of polylines in the wireframe are filled with nurb-surfaces in order to create intermediate and boundary surfaces. Finally, the void spaces completely enclosed by surfaces are labelled in order to define volume identities. In addition, extrusions and different volumetric Boolean operations were used in order to obtain a variety of anatomical shapes. The dimensions and locations of organs and limbs were obtained from 2D medical images. Once the geometry is defined in terms of polylines, nurb-surfaces and volumes, the surfaces of the model are automatically meshed with the advancing front method [123–125]. This approach has been mostly used for creating the H models in Chapters 5 and 6.

The Blender-based approach was mostly used for the pregnant woman model. In this approach, the mesh is created from scratch out of convenient manipulation of primitive objects, such as deformation, inflation, extrusion, etc. Medical images and dimensions from orthogonal points of view were taken in order to build the models.

To the best of the author knowledge, the kind of tools such as Blender [122] are traditionally used in 'artistic' applications, such as character animations. However, their preprocessing capabilities are very appealing for building and manipulating BEM complex meshes, and their use is not commonly spread in mesh generation for engineering applications. One of the reasons may be that these tools are not adequate for FEM type meshes or other numerical approaches which require volume discretisation.

The internal variables of the software can be relatively easily accessed by means of the Python scripting language. This allowed to export meshes and geometrical information for the BEM code developed in this thesis. The versatility and adaptability of this geometry modeller has helped to improve the modelling construction of the woman and to introduce more realistic details in the geometry. Figure A1 shows a view of the blender environment and customisation in order to use it as preprocessor. The GID post-processor and the General Public License (GPL) tool Gmsh [126] were employed for post-processing the results of this work.

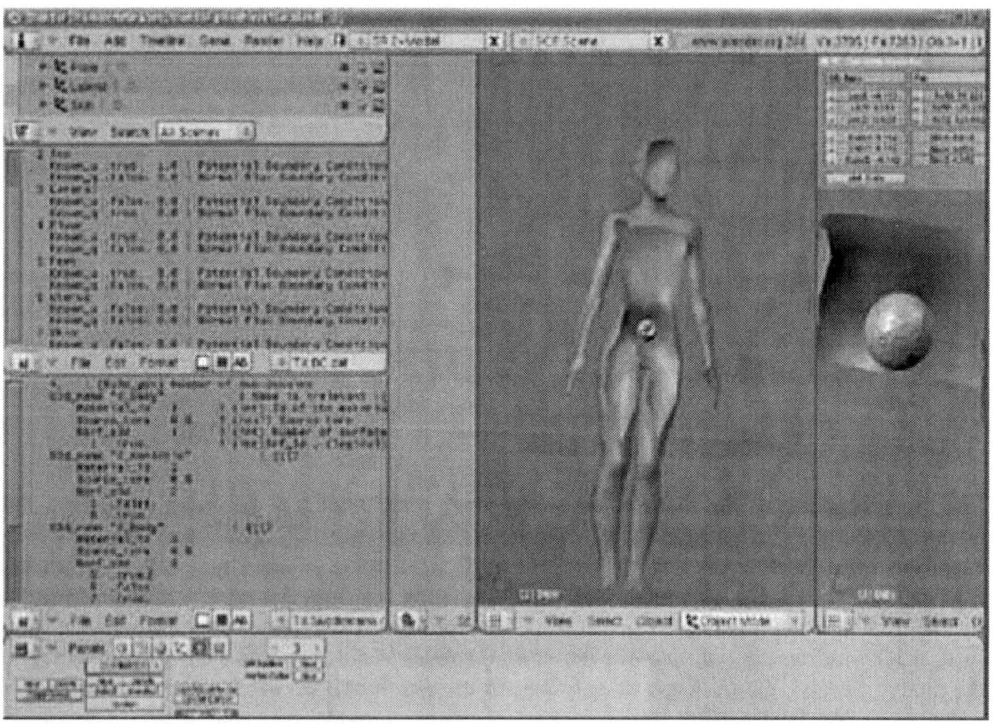

Figure A1: Blender workspace environment.

List of Figures

List of Tables

Symbols and Units

This thesis adopts the SI system of units. The list of basic and derived symbols with their associated units are shown below.

Symbol	Definition	Symbol for unit	In terms of other units	In terms of SI units
C	capacitance	farad F	C/V	$m^{-2}\ kg^{-1}\ s^4\ A^2$
q	charge	coulomb C	$A\ s^{-1}$	$A\ s^{-1}$
G	conductance	Siemens S	Ω^{-1} or A/V	$m^{-2}\ kg^{-1}\ s^3\ A^2$
σ	conductivity	$S\ m^{-1}$	$\Omega^{-1}m^{-1}$	$m^{-3}\ kg^{-1}\ s^3\ A^2$
j	current density		$A\ m^{-2}$	$A\ m^{-2}$
E	EF		$V\ m^{-1}$	$kg\ m\ A^{-1}s^{-3}$
D	EF flux density		$C\ m^{-2}$	$m^{-2}\ A\ s^{-1}$
W	energy	joule J	N m	$m^2\ kg\ s^{-2}$
S	power density	watt m^{-2}	$J\ s^{-1}\ m^{-2}$	$kg\ s^{-3}$
ω	radian frequency	hertz F	Hz	s^{-1}
Z	impedance	ohm	$\Omega\ V^{-1}$	$m^2\ kg\ s^{-3}\ A^{-3}$
L	inductance	henry H	$Wb\ A^{-1}$	$m^2\ kg\ s^{-2}\ A^{-2}$
H	magnetic field	$A\ m^{-1}$	$A\ m^{-1}$	$A\ m^{-1}$
B	magnetic induction	tesla T	$Wb\ m^2$	$kg\ A^{-1}s^{-2}$
μ	permeability	henry m^{-1}	$H\ m^{-1}$	$kg\ m\ A^{-2}\ s^{-2}$
ϵ	permittivity	farad m^{-1}	$F\ m^{-1}$	$kg^{-1}\ m^{-3}\ A^2\ s^4$
P	power	watt W		$J\ s^{-1}\ m^2\ kg\ s^{-3}$
X	reactance	ohm Ω		$m^2\ kg\ s^{-3}\ A^{-2}$
R	resistance	ohm Ω	V/A	$m^2\ kg\ s^{-3}\ A^{-2}$
ρ	resistivity	ohm m	Ω m	$m^3\ kg\ s^{-3}\ A^{-2}$
V	voltage	volt V	W/A	$m^2\ kg\ s^{-3}\ A^{-1}$
ϵ_0	permittivity of vacuum			$8.854 \times 10^{-12}\ F\ m^{-1}$.
μ_0	permeability of vacuum			$1.257 \times 10^{-62}\ H\ m^{-1}$.

Acronyms

BEM	Boundary element method
BIE	Boundary integral equation
CFN	Continuous freedom node
DFN	Discontinuous freedom node
ELF	Extremely low frequency
EM	Electromagnetic
EMC	Electromagnetic compatibility
FD	Finite difference
FDTD	Finite difference time domain
FEM	Finite element method
ICNIRP	International Commission on Non-Ionizing Radiation Protection
S-BEM	Staggered-boundary element method

WITPRESS ...*for scientists by scientists*

Failure Assessment of Thin-walled Structures with Particular Reference to Pipelines

L. ZHANG, Wessex Institute of Technology, UK

This book describes integrity management procedures for thin-walled structures such as gas pipelines. It covers various methods for the analysis of crack growth in thin-walled structures and the probability of failure evaluation of pipelines using the Monte-Carlo simulation.

The focus of this book is on the practical applications of the boundary element method, finite element method and probabilistic fracture mechanics. Popular methods for SIF calculation and crack growth are presented and the evaluation of failure probabilities based on BS7910 is also explained in detail. The procedures described in the book can be used to optimise the maintenance of pipelines, thereby reducing the operating costs. This book will be of interest to pipeline engineers, postgraduate students and university researchers.

ISBN: 978-1-84564-420-8 eISBN: 978-1-84564-421-5
Forthcoming apx 160pp apx £59.00

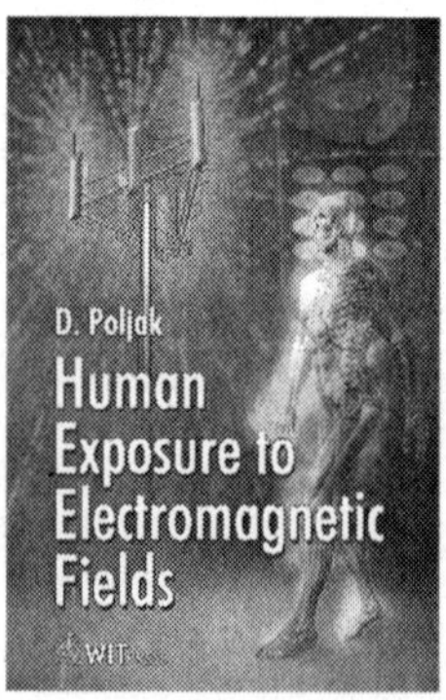

Human Exposure to Electromagnetic Fields

D. POLJAK, University of Split, Croatia

The field of computational bioelectromagnetics has grown rapidly in the last decades, but until now there has not been a comprehensive text on the many aspects of interaction between human beings and electromagnetic fields. This text fills the gap.

Partial Contents: Electrosmog–Environmental Risk of Radiation Pollution; Sources of Electromagnetic Fields and Incident Field Dosimetry; Electromagnetic Modelling of the Human Body; Thermal Modelling of the Human Body; Coupling Mechanisms Between Electromagnetic Fields and the Human Body; Safety Standards and Exposure Limits.

Series: Advances in Electrical and Electronic Engineering, Vol 6
ISBN: 1-85312-997-6
Published 2004 200pp £89.00